08 SEP 1998 WA 90 PAP 14.95

Transcultural care: a guide for health care professionals

Transcultural care:
a guide for health care
professionals

by

Irena Papadopoulos
Mary Tilki
Gina Taylor

Quay
Books

Quay Books, Division of Mark Allen Publishing Limited
Jesses Farm, Snow Hill, Dinton, Nr. Salisbury, Wilts, SP3 5HN

Mark Allen Publishing Ltd, 1998
ISBN 1-85642-051 5

British Library Cataloguing-in-Publications Data
A catalogue record for this book is available from the
BritishLibrary

Printed in Great Britain by Redwood Books,
Trowbridge, Wiltshire

Contents

Preface   vii

Introduction   ix

1. Health of minority ethnic groups by Irena
    Papadopoulos and Jo Alleyne   1

2. Health and citizenship by Gina Taylor   18

3. Old age in Afro-Caribbean and Asian
    communities in Britain by Mary Tilki   44

4. The health needs of the Greek Cypriot people
    living in the UK by Irena Papadopoulos   69

5. The health of the Irish in Britain by Mary Tilki   125

6. Health care for refugees and asylum-seekers in
    Britain by Gina Taylor   152

7. Developing transcultural skills by Irena
    Papadopoulos, Mary Tilki and Gina Taylor   175

8. Conclusion by Gina Taylor, Mary Tilki and
    Irena Papadopoulos   212

Index   225

Preface

This book is intended for health care professionals. As all the authors have a background in nursing and draw heavily on their experiences it is likely that the book will be of most interest to nurses, both pre- and post-registration. We do, however, believe that it will provide a useful consideration of transcultural issues for anyone engaged in health care.

The book has been written because we strongly believe that health care education in general, and nurse education in particular, is failing in any significant way to prepare students to develop knowledge, skills and attitudes relevant to caring for clients from diverse cultures. We offer the reader information concerning the lifestyles and health needs of people from some specific ethnic backgrounds.

It is now more important than ever for health care professionals to understand the wider social, political and economic factors which place individuals and groups at a disadvantage. These factors may affect an individual's access to health care provision.

Almost all recent government reports and health related policies emphasise the centrality of the client at all levels of decision making. This means that the clients' views must be taken into consideration when planning and delivering health care.

If clients are to be empowered to participate in health care decisions, health care professionals need to acquire cultural understanding and must recognise how society creates disadvantage.

It is therefore imperative that professional education responds to this challenge in a positive and practical manner. This book aims to address these challenges by adopting an anti-discriminatory stance which recognises the different forms that discrimination may take, and regards cultural diversity as enriching, both in terms of the educational process and everyday life, rather than as a problem.

Introduction

This book was written in response to a number of reports and health initiatives, such as the *Health of the Nation* (HMSO, 1993), the Patient's Charter, the *Health Policy for Europe* (WHO, 1992), to name but a few. At the same time, it is a response to a variety of international problems which have led to a rapid escalation in the number of migrants, refugees and asylum-seekers requesting refuge in Britain. It is our view that a resurgence of racism is likely to make that refuge a bitter and inhospitable experience for many. It is also important to acknowledge that these ethnic and racial groups in Britain have traditionally been less successful in gaining access to health care than the indigenous population; further, some of their needs have been neglected (Henley, 1982; Hopkins and Bahl, 1993).

Law (1996) argues that, although local authorities and social services departments adopted a range of anti-racist policies in the 70s and 80s, the NHS was impervious to anti-racist and multiculturalist ideas until quite recently. He suggests that insularity from such ideas originated in tenets of professional and clinical freedom which resisted attention to the specific needs of minority ethnic groups in the belief that professionals knew best. Medical autonomy with little client or community participation and the absence of frameworks for public accountability meant there was no real pressure to consider culture or ethnicity. Community health councils may not have been particularly representative of minority groups but their marginalisation following the health reforms of the 1980s reduced public accountability even further. The removal of local authority representatives on NHS trust boards in the 1990s further reduced opportunities for local influence, which particularly affected areas with a high proportion of minority ethnic groups. The commitment to challenge racism was not incorporated in statutory duties for the National Health Service as it was for public bodies, such as the Housing Corporation. In 1992, the Commission for Racial Equality (CRE) launched the *Code of Practice in Primary Health Care Services* which was endorsed by ministers without parliamentary approval. It was evident in May 1993 that fewer than thirty of the six hundred authorities intended to implement the code (Law, 1996). Despite these weaknesses, Blakemore and Drake (1996) suggest that the NHS reforms and the new managerialism could afford opportunities for fairer and better provision.

Smaje (1995) comments on the continuing debate between multiculturalism and anti-racism. Whereas multiculturalism tends to emphasise the existence of different cultural traditions in contemporary Britain and promotes tolerance and understanding, anti-racism places a more political emphasis on the forces that structure and determine access to power in society. The model of transcultural care offered in this book proposes that these two approaches can be combined in a contructive way.

While various textbooks have raised awareness and increased understanding of the needs of specific cultural groups (Mares *et al,* 1985), the centrality of racism has not been fully debated (Alleyne *et al,* 1994). Thus, while certain chapters of this book do offer information concerning the cultural backgrounds of groups who have received little attention in previous literature, an attempt is also made to move beyond description to take an anti-discriminatory stance and identify the effects of racism on health. Inequalities, in terms of ethnic group, do not occur in isolation, so it is important to remember that other variables such as social class, age and gender also need to be taken into consideration. For example, a refugee will belong to a certain ethnic group but may also be homeless and unemployed. It has been acknowledged that people in the lower occupational classes have worse health than those in higher classes; there are also differences in the health experiences of men and women. Thus, when a member of a minority ethnic group is located within his/her socio-economic position, it is possible to appreciate the similarities that might exist with members of the indigenous population in a similar socio-economic position.

With these concerns in mind, and while acknowledging the existence of a multitude of minority ethnic groups, only certain groups have been selected for attention in this book as a result of either the personal or professional experiences of the authors with the groups concerned, and a desire and a sense of obigation to share those experiences. The aim is thus to add to the growing literature about transcultural care and also to locate the issues within the context of the ever popular concept of citizenship.

The World Health Organisation's *Health Policy for Europe* (1992) aims to reduce inequalities in health both within and between countries. Promotion of health and prevention of disease will be considered through the medium of a participating community. Such an approach is the essence of citizenship but questions are raised concerning who is included and who is excluded from such participation. It is argued that poor health can pose a barrier to becoming an active member of any community and so reduce any individual's opportunities for participating in community health initiatives. Ahmad (1993) argues that health and ill health are socially produced and are mediated by an individual's citizenship status, that is, their degree of inclusion or exclusion in society.

Citizenship has traditionally been discussed in terms of cultural homogeneity, but given the pluralistic nature of contemporary British society, cultural homogeneity can no longer form a foundation for citizenship (Oliver and Heater, 1994).

Chapter 1: explores the health of minority ethnic groups. It addresses ethnic monitoring and examines the evidence of racism in the NHS. Finally it discusses the components of care necessary to provide individualised and culturally competent care.

Chapter 2: explores citizenship and its relation to health.

Chapter 3: considers the needs of older people from the Afro-Caribbean and Asian communities living in Britain.

Chapter 4: reports the results of a survey on the lifestyles and health needs of Greek Cypriots living in Britain. Literature on the health needs of this ethnic group is practically non-existent; this chapter is a unique contribution on this topic.

Chapter 5: looks at the health of Irish people living in Britain. It provides a useful insight into the patterns of Irish migration and discusses the prevalence of certain diseases within this group.

Chapter 6: concerns the plight of refugees and asylum-seekers in Britain. It addresses the health problems which may arise and also describes a local health education project involving members of refugee groups.

Chapter 7: proposes a model for transcultural care and offers examples of situations drawn from the experiences of the authors. Consideration of the issues raised by these examples should assist the reader to acquire and develop skills to enhance caring encounters with members of diverse cultural groups.

We do not suggest that it would be possible for professional carers to acquire a working knowledge of the way of life of every cultural group that they may encounter, but we hope that this chapter will facilitate the development of skills that the practitioner can use to learn from his/her clients.

Resources to assist in the acquisition of culturally competent skills, are listed. These include resources from the 'arts' embracing popular literature and films, as we firmly believe that in the era of lifelong learning it is important to be aware of the vast resources that surround us in everyday life and that can inform the everyday work of any carer. For example, while the theme of AIDS sufferers is not addressed in this volume, the celebrated film *Philadelphia* is recommended as valuable viewing in order to foster reflection on discrimination in practice. This is in keeping with our belief that there are lessons that can be learned from experience with one particular disadvantaged group which can be transferred to another.

Twine (1994) argues that societal messages of low worth and stigmatisation damage self identity and affect health behaviour. It is vital, therefore, that those engaged in health care are alert to, and take steps to address, such messages directed at disadvantaged groups or 'second class citizens' because of age, class, race, gender or a combination of all these.

The final chapter attempts to bring together the major concepts and concerns covered in the previous chapters.

The World Health Organisation Regional Office for Europe (1992) notes that among the possible trends in a future Europe are increased migration both from outside Europe and within, and widening differences between parts of Europe and between socio-economic groups; though it has also been noted that society may evolve to become more responsible and caring.

The European Union has declared 1997 the European Year Against Racism. The success of the events which have take place during the year, should contribute towards the reduction (hopefully the elimination) of discrimination in all forms, not only in terms of race, but also in terms of people's backgrounds, beliefs and lifestyles. In short, an end to intolerance of any sort.

It is our belief that working towards improving the health and so the life chances of disadvantaged groups of people, will make for a better society for all to live in.

References

Ahmad WIU (ed.) (1993) *Race and Health in Contemporary Britain.* Open University Press, Buckingham

Alleyne J, Papadopoulos I, Tilki M (1994) Antiracism within transcultural nurse education. Transcultural Care Series. *Br J Nurs* **3**(12): 635–7

Blakemore K, Drake R (1996) *Understanding Equal Opportunity Policies.* Prentice Hall Europe, Hemel Hempstead

Commission for Racial Equality (1992) *Race Relations Code of Practice in Primary Health Care Services.* CRE, London

Henley A (1982) *The Asian Patient in Hospital and Home.* King Edward Hospital Fund for London

Hopkins A, Bahl V (eds.) (1993) *Access to Health Care for People from Black and Ethnic Minorities.* RCP, London

Law I (1996) *Racism Ethnicity and Social Policy.* Prentice Hall Europe, Hemel Hempstead

Mares P, Henley A, Baxter C (1985) *Health Care in Multiracial Britain.* Health Education Council and the National Extension College, Cambridge

Oliver D, Heater D (1994) *The Foundations of Citizenship.* Harester Wheatsheaf, London

Smaje C (1995) *Health, 'Race' and Ethnicity. Making Sense of the Evidence.* King's Fund Institute, London

Twine F (1994) *Citizenship and Social Rights. The Interdependence of self and society.* Sage, London

World Health Organisation Regional Office for Europe (1992) *Targets for Health for All: The Health Policy for Europe. Summary of the updated edition.* WHO Regional Office for Europe, Copenhagen

1

Health of minority ethnic groups

Irena Papadopoulos and Jo Alleyne

Background

It is widely accepted that Britain has been, is, and will continue to be a multicultural, multi-ethnic and multiracial society. There are an estimated three million people of ethnic minority origin residing in England and Wales, constituting 6% of the total population (OPCS, 1992). It is also true to say that minority ethnic groups within this society suffer from disadvantages and discriminatory practices within the health care system (Baxter C, 1988(b); Torkington, 1992; Ahmad, 1993; Jamdagni, 1996). Furthermore, the preparation of health care practitioners has yet to meet the challenge of delivering effective and appropriate health care that meets the needs of ethnic minority groups (Papadopoulos *et al*, 1995).

Despite the fact that our understanding of health and illness has to be considered in terms of social and cultural determinants and not just biological factors, there is as yet little evidence to suggest that the education of health care professionals explores ethnic health in any meaningful and substantial way. It seems that we have a long way to go before we can achieve the *Health of the Nation's* requirement for such professionals to address the needs of black and ethnic minority groups and to take positive steps to eliminate discrimination. This requirement is reinforced by the Chief Medical Officer's report *On the State of the Public Health 1991* (Calman, 1992), which points out that people working within the health services should be aware of ethnic differences in disease patterns, and that they should consider how such differences can be responded to by the provision of appropriate services that embrace all aspects of health care and by new approaches that take account of cultural variations.

It can be argued that the relative inaction of the health care professions in addressing the needs of minority ethnic groups results from a want of definition of the most commonly used terms within the literature, or from lack of commitment to providing individualised care or even that it is due to racism. While this chapter does not attempt to provide a detailed analysis of the various concepts in common use, such as culture, race, ethnicity, ethnocentricity, racism, discrimination and transcultural nursing, it is important to define these terms, as some, if not all, are often used interchangeably, either in a meaningless way or in order to conceal racism (*Table 1.1*).

Table 1.1: Useful definitions

culture	the shared way of life of a group of people (Berry JW *et al,* 1992). It includes those ideas, techniques and habits passed by one generation to another a social heritage
race	characterised by physical appearance, determined by ancestry and perceived as a permanent genetic state (Fernando, 1991)
ethnicity	the basis for defining groups of people who feel themselves to be separate in multiracial and multicultural societies. It implies a sense of belonging (Fernando, 1991)
ethno-centricity	the tendency to use one's own group's standards as *the* standard, when viewing other groups to place one's group at the top of a hierarchy and to rank all others lower (Sumner, 1906)
racism	a doctrine or ideology or dogma. It is recognised by the behaviour of individuals and institutions based on concepts of racial difference (Fernando, 1991)

Fernando (1991) offers an enlightening analysis of the above terms and suggests that race, culture and ethnicity are interrelated in complex ways depending on historical, political and social factors. The choice of term by which a particular group is described generally depends on the style and degree of racism in the society at the time, the extent to which people in power appreciate the situation, and the particular purpose for which classification by race, ethnicity or culture is required. Fernando summarises his analysis of the concepts of race, culture and ethnicity in *Table 1.2*

Table 1.2: Characteristics, determinants and perceptions of race, culture and ethnicity.

	characterised by	determined by	perceived as
race	physical appearance	genetic ancestry	permanent (genetic/ biological)
culture	behaviour attitudes	upbringing choice	changeable (assimilation, acculturation)
ethnicity	sense of belonging group identity	social pressures psychological need	partially changeable

Smaje (1995) reminds us that discriminatory behaviour can result from direct racism, from indirect or institutional racism and from ethno-centrism, although these distinctions should not be overemphasised: it is the lack of power to contest majority assumptions and prejudices that lends racism its force in many people's experience of health care.

Ahmad (1993) states that the world of ethnicity and health is divided between those favouring a culturalist approach and, more recently, those who focus on structural factors. The former ignore considerations of power and structural aspects of culture, the latter have sacrificed culture on the altar of anti-racism. In nursing, a culturalist approach has been promoted mainly by Leininger through her work on transcultural nursing, which she defined more than ten years ago as:

a humanistic and scientific area of formal study and practice in nursing which is focused upon the comparative study of cultures with regard to differences and similarities in care, health, and illness patterns, based upon cultural values, beliefs, and practices of different cultures in the world, and the use of this knowledge to provide culturally-specific and/or universal nursing care to people (1984, 42).

During the past three decades Leininger and her associates and students have researched more than 50 cultures and have identified 173 care constructs. Leininger has developed a theory of nursing called 'culture care diversity and universality'. The theory comes complete with a conceptual framework called the 'sunrise model' and a qualitative research methodology called 'ethnonursing'. Within the theory, the aims of nursing are defined as cultural care preservation/maintenance, cultural care accommodation/negotiation, and cultural care repatterning/restructuring. Leininger's ultimate aspiration is that,

> *someday all people in the world will be served by professional nurses prepared in transcultural nursing and using research findings generated from Culture Care theory.* (p417)

Leininger's work is not without its critics. Tripp-Reimer and Dougherty (1985) criticise transcultural nursing for apparent lack of rigour in the research studies which are qualitative in nature. Bruni (1988), on the other hand, believes that it is not enough to focus on the culture itself: factors that influence the culture such as poverty and racism must be considered, a view echoed by Sands and Hale (1988) and Alleyne *et al* (1994). Ahmad (1993) argues that there is no reason why research, writing or practice cannot encompass a sophisticated conception of culture well located in its socio-economic, political and historical context.

Racism in the NHS

It is widely acknowledged that discrimination exists at every level of the health service, affecting nurses, other health care workers and clients (Beishon *et al,* 1995). The form that this discrimination takes varies, from deterring young people from black and minority ethnic groups from entering the health care professions, to the provision of irrelevant health care (Allen, 1991). The current health care system fails many of its users, notably those who are not white or middle class (Torkington, 1992). At best these groups are received with indifference, but many are exposed to neglect and also hostility to their culture (Torkington, 1984). Some find their problems trivialised, while in other cases misdiagnosis occurs (Francis *et al,* 1989).

A cursory examination of the education of all health professionals reveals a recent move towards the introduction of the 'multicultural' model, which emphasises the need for a better understanding of the customs, traditions and religious activities of minority ethnic groups. Karmi (1992) asserts that this change is long overdue as there is a widespread ignorance among health professionals at all levels about the culture and customs of the ethnic patients they encounter. Kushnick (1988) argues that well-meaning attempts to correct the deficiencies in knowledge and practice that have been reported within a multicultural framework can be counterproductive, since they may reinforce stereotypes of ethnic differences. It is not surprising that many professionals and authors strongly recommend that education and practice should move from this model to one which focuses on anti-racism (Ahmad, 1993; Stubbs, 1993; Papadopoulos *et al*, 1995). Health professionals must attempt to challenge racism and avoid approaches that are merely confined to the reiteration of culture. It is naïve to suppose that multiculturalist approaches can become anti-racist, as anti-racist approaches involve a more radical restructuring of racist systems. In nursing, 'transcultural education' has been defined as both the promotion of understanding of the diverse lifestyles, beliefs and values of our clients and, at the same time, the promotion of anti-racism (Papadopoulos *et al*, 1994; Alleyne *et al*, 1994). It is essential that we develop a body of knowledge for health care students that provides insights into cultural and ethnic issues whilst also addressing the multi-faceted nature of racism.

The need for information on clients' ethnicity

In April 1995, 'ethnic group' became a mandatory field in the contract minimum data set for admitted patient care in England, which includes in-patients and day case patients.

As discussed in the previous sections of this chapter, there is a growing concern that people with different racial and cultural backgrounds show different patterns of disease and have different health service needs. Furthermore, it is well documented that black and minority ethnic groups are less likely to find health services that are 'appropriate, accessible, adequate and accountable' (NAHA, 1988).

In 1994 the NHS Executive announced, in the document produced as guidance on implementing ethnic group data collection, that the classification and coding of ethnic groups will continue to be based on that used in the 1991 OPCS census. These are: White, Black Caribbean, Black African, Black other, Indian, Pakistani, Bangladeshi, Chinese, Other Ethnic Group.

The same source defines 'ethnic group' as a group of people who share characteristics such as language, history, culture, upbringing, religion, nationality, and geographical and ancestral origins and place, thus providing the group with a distinct identity as seen both by themselves and others. It is important at this point to distinguish between the terms 'ethnic group' and 'ethnic or racial origin'. 'Ethnic group', is the term currently being used within the NHS; it refers to the individuals' own perception of themselves in response to all the cultural and other factors that define ethnic group. 'Ethnic origin' is used in medicine to describe the genetic make-up of a person. Self classification is a fundamental principle underpinning the collection of ethnic group data. It is important because the way people regard themselves influences their behaviour. In addition, classification by someone else is unreliable and unrepresentative.

It is hoped that through the availability of patient ethnic group data the NHS will provide better health care by making sure that all sectors of the community have equal access to the services provided, and that they receive more effective care and more efficient discharge arrangements.

Assessing health care needs for minority ethnic groups

In the past 20 years a variety of approaches to needs assessment has reflected a variety of historical concerns. The period of rational planning in the 1970s left a legacy of comprehensive reviews of services arguably taking the place of any pragmatic attempt to bring about change. In the 1980s the focus of attention was on the differences between locality, which, although useful for the allocation of funding, had little to say about the type and level of services actually required. By contrast, the agenda for needs assessment in the late 1990s is about defining the nature and level of services required to care for and improve the health of the population (DoH, 1991), using a variety of approaches in data collection, for example, epidemiological returns, surveys, focus groups, qualitative studies, case studies and so on. In the document *Assessing health care needs* (DoH, 1991), 'need' is defined as 'the population's ability to benefit from health care'. Ethnic monitoring is a major initiative that aims to contribute to the assessment of health needs. Ethnic monitoring will provide quantitative information that must be complemented by qualitative information about the various ethnic groups. The *Health of the Nation Strategy* (DoH, 1992) requires the needs of people from black and minority ethnic groups to be considered when addressing the key areas (coronary heart disease and stroke, cancers, mental illness, HIV/AIDS and sexual health, accidents). In addition the *Health of the Nation Strategy* reiterates that the National Health Service reforms provide an opportunity for the health of black and minority ethnic groups to become part of the mainstream of healthcare delivery.

Health authorities are required to assess the health needs of the local population in order to purchase appropriate health services locally. The NHS reforms have also highlighted the need for appropriate community consultation, as black and minority ethnic groups have not been sufficiently involved in giving their opinion on local health services in the past. This reflects the new mood within the health services, which Mohammed (1993) described as promoting the value of the user and the community in general. All this is a far cry from the secrecy and limited consultation for which the Health Service has been noted.

The growing interest in the role of users in the development of services has been reiterated in a number of government and Department of Health initiatives such as the Citizen's Charter and its health counterpart the Patient's Charter. Clearly the attempt to assess the health needs of the population more efficiently is closely linked with the aspiration of the NHS to provide quality services for all. This purpose is articulated in the guidance for the 1996/7 priorities and planning issued by the NHSE in 1995. The medium term priorities are:

- to work towards the development of a primary care-led NHS, in which decisions about the purchasing and provision of health care are taken as close to patients as possible

- in partnership with local authorities, to purchase and monitor a comprehensive range of secure, residential, in-patient and community services to enable people with mental illness to receive effective care and treatment in the most appropriate setting in accordance with their needs

• to improve the cost effectiveness of services throughout the NHS, and thereby secure the greatest health gain from the resources available, through formulating decisions on the basis of appropriate evidence about clinical effectiveness

• to give greater influence to users of NHS services and their carers over their own care, the development and definition of standards set for NHS services locally and the development of NHS policy both locally and nationally

• to ensure, in collaboration with local authorities and other organisations, that integrated services are in place to meet needs for continuing health care and to allow elderly, disabled or vulnerable people to be supported in the community

• to develop NHS organisations as good employers with particular reference to workforce planning, education and training, employment policy and practice, the development of teamwork, rewards systems, staff utilisation and staff welfare

In seeking to achieve its purpose as a public service, the NHS aims to judge its results under three headings: equity, efficiency and esponsiveness. This cannot be achieved if the NHS lacks information about 6% of its clients. Bahl (1993) stated that lack of adequate information on black and ethnic minority populations meant that fewer services were planned in a sensitive manner. This led the Department to take initiatives such as ethnic monitoring to improve the health of minority groups. The key themes in the development of these health policies are:

• elimination of racial discrimination

• availability of data on black and ethnic minority groups

• delivery of appropriate quality services

• training of health professionals

• information for black and ethnic minority groups on health and health services

• recognition of differing patterns of health and disease

The need for individualised care: lessons from nursing

The consensus of opinion in the world of nursing, over the last thirty years, has been that nursing practice has needed to shift from a reductionist approach to an approach that emphasised the needs of the individual as a whole. In Britain this shift was embraced at the level of attempting to move from a task orientated approach to a nursing process approach, which was considered the ideal vehicle for delivering individualised care. There has been an unquestioning assumption that this approach has been accepted and is now in practice.

This chapter challenges this assumption by proposing to redefine some of the original claims in light of the recognition that Britain is a culturally and ethnically diverse society, a fact to which the earlier British nursing theorists, such as Roper *et al (*1990), gave only minimal attention. It is our belief that this omission needs to be rectified and be added to the current discussion about the challenges facing nursing practice in the 21st century as outlined by the Heathrow Debate (DoH, 1994). We believe that there is a need for an enhanced transcultural framework in order to promote individualised care. The word 'enhanced' is introduced here to differentiate from the definition and theory expounded by Leininger discussed in a previous section of this chapter. Our 'enhanced transcultural framework' combines the need for cultural knowledge with the need to address anti-racism. We shall also consider the importance of the nurse–client relationship and mutual communication for effective nursing care. The findings from our recently completed study on teaching transcultural care will be drawn from to illustrate the failure of nursing education to promote culturally sensitive and anti-racist care.

The *Delphi Survey of optimum practice in nursing, midwifery and health visiting* (University of Manchester, 1993), suggested that optimum practice should be aimed at what the clients need and not what the practitioner thinks they want. While not disagreeing with the sentiments expressed in this survey, we are nevertheless concerned that no acknowledgement is made of culturally specific needs of clients. Furthermore, this failure to locate nursing practice within an enhanced transcultural framework prevents individualised care from becoming a reality. Evidence for this is provided by a recent report from the King's Fund (1990) which has questioned the ability of nurses and midwives to deliver adequate and appropriate health care to Britain's multiracial and multicultural population. In addition, the Audit Commission's report (1992) stated that patients in general received little individualised care, whilst earlier evidence suggests that patients from minority ethnic groups are additionally disadvantaged (Alleyne and Thomas, 1994; Smaje, 1995).

It is worth noting that the Delphi Survey stated that patient care is only as good as the nurse who provides it and that good patient care comes from a nurse who is motivated, happy at work, has good communication skills, possesses the relevant nursing knowledge, is open to new ideas and is willing to question and change practice as required. These are some of the areas also identified by Murphy and Macleod-Clark (1993) as being problematic for nurses when caring for clients from minority ethnic groups. This study highlighted the victim-blaming approach that the nurses adopted. These nurses made no attempt to develop cultural knowledge, skills or attitudes that would have resulted in a less frustrating and more satisfactory experience for the patients.

The nurse–client relationship

It is our belief that appropriate and sensitive, rather than 'good', patient care is dependent on a nurse–client relationship based on mutual respect and trust, which can only be achieved through knowledge and understanding of our clients' cultures and an appreciation of their struggles for equity and dignity, which, as Ahmad (1993) explains, have been part of the history of black and minority ethnic groups. The findings of our research (Papadopoulos *et al,* 1995) suggest that educators are failing to recognise that lack of attention to culturally specific needs is likely to result in inferior or ineffective care. Furthermore, they are also failing adequately to prepare practitioners to provide culturally sensitive care. The majority of our informants admitted that they were not confident of their competence to teach culturally relevant concepts and issues. Our findings also highlighted the fact that little attention is paid to the importance of health beliefs and the impact these have on behaviour in health and illness. Omissions of this kind will obviously limit the extent to which care is planned and negotiated with clients. They suggest that conflicts may well occur between clients and nurses if their health beliefs are incongruent.

The concept of partnership is now established in British nursing literature as a desirable characteristic of the nurse–patient relationship (Pearson and Vaughan, 1986; McMahon and Pearson, 1991). The RCN (1987) *Position Statement on Nursing* stated:

Each patient has a right to be a partner in his own care-planning and receive relevant information, support and encouragement from the nurse which will permit him to make informed choices and become involved in his own care.

This position will not be achieved while nurses are unable to understand the needs of clients from a diversity of cultures.

Mutual communication

Another essential element for the development of a nurse–client relationship that is fundamental to optimum practice and individualised care is the ability to communicate effectively with clients from different cultural backgrounds. Communication is an essential element of all nursing models; nurses often identify language barriers as communication problems but invariably fail to deal adequately with them apart from involving interpreters. While acknowledging the important service that interpreters provide and the assistance that relatives can offer, it is our belief that nurses are in a unique position to offer creative solutions to meet their clients' communication needs. Computer technology, for example, has made it possible for people travelling abroad to use cheap and easily accessible pocket translators. It should not be beyond the realms of possibility for nurses to collaborate with computer experts in order to devise appropriate phrases in different languages for such pocket devices, which would greatly enhance the ability of nurses and clients to communicate. While we are waiting for this development, nurses could create their own lists of useful phrases on cards for easy use. These could be combined with symbols and pictures similar to those used by the Maketon alphabet (signs and pictures used to communicate with people with learning difficulties) in order to improve communication.

It is our view that failure to communicate is unacceptable in current nursing practice. It is unrealistic and inadequate for nurse educators and practitioners to exempt themselves from providing culturally congruent care, to the extent that Cortese (1990) claims it to be an example of unethical practice. In order to overcome these challenges, practitioners must start by demonstrating commitment to mutual communication. Kavanagh and Kennedy (1992) propose that commitment to mutual communication is based on the following assumptions:

- the recognition and value of human dignity

- cultural relativism as an acceptable and preferred condition

- willingness to alter personal behaviour in response to the communication process

- willingness to decrease personal resistance and defensiveness

There is a tendency to cite dialects and speaking styles, such as that of the British born Afro-Caribbean youth or the use of jargon within a professional group, as barriers to effective communication. Pedersen (1988) suggests that it is crucial for practitioners to be able to recognise and deal with cross-cultural communication; otherwise there is a risk of misleading assessments and inappropriate care. Effective cross-cultural communication requires awareness that communication is possible even though mistakes may occur; it also requires sensitivity to the communication process, knowledge of the clients' communication styles and a set of practice skills.

Culturally specific knowledge

Another important element needed to promote individualised care is knowledge. Our recent research has indicated that it is unrealistic for nurses to be expected to address the needs of the many different cultural groups they may encounter. Furthermore, our research indicated that there is a dearth of culturally specific knowledge available to inform professional health carers. However, our evidence suggests that, even in cases where knowledge does exist, teachers are reluctant to make use of it, primarily because of the fear of creating stereotypes. Despite this, teachers do have a responsibility to ensure that students become informed about cultural issues affecting health; there is no evidence to suggest that stereotyping will occur. In contrast, Foolchand (1995) advocates the exploration of stereotypes within the context of race and ethnicity as a vital component of the curriculum. In addition, the majority of teachers claimed that the principles of individualised client care more than adequately dealt with all client needs, including cultural needs, thus rejecting the use of culturally specific knowledge (Papadopoulos *et al,* 1995). It is highly questionable that such an approach, without the existence of a body of culturally specific knowledge, could be translated into culturally sensitive care. We would go so far as to state that health professionals have an obligation to do precisely what they are avoiding, if only in response to the statements and standards for practice from the Department of Health (1991) and the UKCC (1992).

Open to new ideas

It is clear that a great deal needs to be done to equalise the relationship between practitioners and clients in order that optimum nursing care can be achieved. To achieve this, nurses must be able to adopt new ideas, be reflexive and reflective, and be forward thinking and innovative. This position supports Pedersen's (1988) claim that caring for individuals from diverse cultures requires the continual testing of stereotypes against reality and the modification of interaction according to the available evidence.

Cultural awareness and sensitivity imply learning to recognise when old information no longer applies. Nurses, along with all other providers of services across the health and social care sector, must ensure that wherever they can, they clarify what works, import this information to those who need it and reflect it in practice. Effectiveness will increasingly be the key to recognition. Research based knowledge must underpin and inform nursing practice (DoH, 1994).

It could be argued that the best way to learn about the cultural background of the client is to ask him or her. While that is a desirable starting point for any nurse–client interaction, it is important to bear in mind that this approach cannot replace knowledge which could precede client encounters and which could develop during pre- and post-registration education and personal development. Learning from clients is itself an innovation. However, this may not always be possible or appropriate, as, for example in the case of a client who is acutely ill or unconscious. In these situations, the nurse will act in the best interest of the client using sets of assumptions. While there is no guarantee that these assumptions will help her/him plan and deliver individualised care, it could be argued that a nurse who is committed to culturally sensitive care will be more likely to deliver optimum care in comparison with another nurse who lacks this sensitivity and knowledge.

Conclusion

Leddy and Pepper (1989) remind us that the basic moral concern of nursing is with the welfare of other humans. Service to people involves ethical responsibility. Service to society also requires assurances that practitioners are competent. The time has come to address the question: are nurses competent to provide culturally sensitive care? We have argued elsewhere (Papadopoulos *et al*, 1994) that the existing evidence suggests that this is far from being achieved or demonstrated. We have also proposed that a transcultural approach to nursing education and practice will help improve the individualised care given to all clients irrespective of their cultural backgrounds. Cortis (1993) stated that anthropologists have frequently pointed out that by studying and learning from other cultural groups we become more conscious of our own culture. Cultural factors are one of the major forces that influence the quality of health and nursing care. If nursing fails to consider these factors, then it is failing to provide individualised care to all its clients. This is a frightening thought if we begin to contemplate the implications of this statement; we may discover that we cannot hide behind the veil of individualised patient care any longer.

References

Ahmad WIU (ed.) (1993) *Race and Health in Contemporary Britain.* Open University Press, Buckingham

Allen D (1991) From plasters to poverty. *Nur Standard.* **6**(5):18

Alleyne J, Papadopoulos I, Tilki M (1994) Anti-Racism within transcultural education. *B J Nurs* **3**(12):635–7

Alleyne J, Thomas V (1994) The management of sickle cell crisis pain as experienced by patients and their carers. *J Adv Nurs* **19**:725–2

Audit Commission (1992) *Making Time for Patients.* HMSO, London

Bahl V (1993) Development of black and minority health policy at the Department of Health. In: Hopkins A, Bahl V (eds) *Access to Health Care for People from Black and Ethnic Minorities.* RCPL, London

Baxter C (1988b) *The Black Nurse: An Endangered Species. A Case for Equal Opportunities in Nursing.* Training in Health and Race, London

Beishon S *et al* (1995) *Nursing in a Multi-Ethnic NHS.* Policy Studies Institute, London

Berry JW *et al* (1992) *Cross-cultural psychology. Research and Applications.* Cambridge University Press

Bruni N (1988) A critical analysis of transcultural theory. *Australian J Adv Nurs.* **15**(3):26–36

Calam KC (1992) *On the State of Public Health 1991.* HMSO, London

Cortese A (1990) *Ethnic Ethics: The Restructuring of Moral Theory.* The State University of New York Press, Albany

Cortis JD (1993) Transcultural nursing: Appropriateness for Britain. *J Adv in Health and Nursing Care.* **2**(4):67–77

A Delphi Survey of Optimum Practice in Nursing, Midwifery and Health Visiting (1993) The University of Manchester

Department of Health (1991) *Patient's Charter.* HMSO, London

Department of Health: NHS Management Executive (1991) *Assessing Health Care Needs.* HMSO, London

Department of Health (1992) *The Health of the Nation. A Strategy for Health in England.* HMSO, London

Department of Health (1994) *The Challenges for Nursing and Midwifery in the 21st Century. The Heathrow Debate.* HMSO, London

Fernando S (1991) *Mental Health, Race and Culture.* Macmillan in association with Mind Publications, London

Foolchand MK (1995) Promoting racial equality in the nursing curriculum. *Nur Educ Today.* **15**:101–5

Francis E *et al* (1989) Black people and psychiatry in the UK. *Psychiatric Bulletin.* **13**:482–5

Jamdagni L (1996) Race against time. *The Health Services Journal.* **106**(5493): 30–1

Karmi G (ed.) (1992) *The Ethnic Health Factfile: A guide for health professionals who care for people from ethnic minorities.* North West/North East Thames RHAs, London

Kavanagh KH, Kennedy PH (1992) *Promoting Cultural Diversity. Strategies for Health Care Professionals.* Sage, Newbury Park

King Edward's Hospital Fund for London (1990) *Racial Equality: the Nursing Profession.* Task Force Position Paper. Equal Opportunities Task Force Occasional Paper No6, London

Kushnick L (1988) Racism, the National Health Service and the health of black people. *International Journal of Health Services.* **18**: 28–9

Leddy S, Pepper JM (1989) *Conceptual Bases of Professional Nursing* 2nd edn. Lippincott, Philadelphia

Leininger MM (ed.) (1991) *Culture Care, Diversity and Universality: a theory of nursing.* NLN Press, New York

Leininger MM (1984) Transcultural nursing: an essential knowledge and practice field for today. *Canadian Nurse* Dec:41–57

McMahon R , Pearson A (1991) *Nursing as Therapy.* Chapman and Hall, London

Mohamed S (1993) *User-Sensitive Purchasing.* King's Fund Centre, London.

Murphy K, Macleod Clark J (1993) Nurses' experiences of caring for ethnic minority clients. *J Adv Nurs* **18**: 442–50

NAHA (1988) *Action not Words: A strategy to improve health services for black and minority ethnic groups.* NAHA, Birmingham

Doh (1994) *Collecting Ethnic Group Date for Admitted Patient Care. Implemention Guidance and Training Material.* HMSO, London

DoH (1995) *Priorities and planning guidance for the NHS: 1996/97.* HMSO, London.

Papadopoulos I, Tilki M, Alleyne J (1994) Transcultural nursing and nurse education. *Br J Nurs.* **3**(11): 583–6

Papadopoulos I, Alleyne J, Tilki M (1995) *Teaching Transcultural Care: An investigation into the teaching methods suitable for transcultural education for nurses and midwives.* Faculty of Health Studies. Middlesex University

Pearson A, Vaughan B (1986) *Nursing Models for Practice.* Heinemann, London

Pedersen P (1988) The three stages of multicultural development: Awareness, knowledge, and skill. In: Pedersen P ed. *A handbook for developing multicultural awareness.* American Association for Counselling Development Alexandria, VA

Royal College of Nursing (1987) *Position Statement on Nursing.* RCN, London.

Roper N, Logan WW, Tierney A (1990) *The Elements of Nursing: a Model for Nursing Based on a Model for Living* 3rd edn. Churchill Livingstone, Edinburgh

Sands R, Hale S (1988) Enhancing cultural sensitivity in clinical practice. *J Nat Bl Nur Assoc.* **2**(1): 54–63

Smaje C (1995) *Health 'Race' and Ethnicity. Making Sense of the Evidence.* King's Fund Institute, London

Stubbs P (1993) 'Ethnically sensitive' or 'anti-racist'? Models for health research and service delivery. In: Ahmad WIU ed. *Race and Health in Contemporary Britain.* Open University Press, Buckingham

Sumner WR (1906) *Folkways.* Ginn, New York

Torkington P (1983) *The Racial Politics of Health. A Liverpool Profile.* Merseyside Area Profile Group, Department of Sociology, University of Liverpool

Torkington P (1984) The racist and sexist delivery of the NHS- the experience of Black women. In: O'Sullivan S ed. (1987) *Women's Health, A Spare Rib Reader.* Pandora, London

Torkington P (1992) *Black Health; a Political Issue.* Catholic Association for Racial Justice, Liverpool

Tripp-Reimer T, Dougherty M (1985) Cross-cultural nursing research. *Annual Review of Nursing Research.* **3**: 77–104

United Kingdom Central Council for Nursing, Midwifery and Health Visiting (1992) *Code of Conduct for the Nurse, Midwife and Health Visitor.* 3rd edition. UKCC, London

2

Health and citizenship

Gina Taylor

'Citizenship is emerging as the political buzz word of the 1990s' (Plant and Barry, 1990). A glance through the papers reveals a number of headlines that include the word:

> *Citizenship and user-involvement in health provision.* (Senior Nurse)

> *Strangers, citizens and the siege mentality.* (The European)

> *£1m plan to turn neighbours from hell into model citizens.* (Sunday Times)

> *How MEPs would build a house fit for their citizens.* (The European)

> *The citizens are always right.* (Guardian Society)

This chapter concerns the relationship between citizenship and health. It supports Ahmad's (1993) statement that health and ill health are socially produced and mediated by an individual's citizenship status.

The concept of citizenship

What does citizenship mean? The concept of citizenship may be traced as far back as Ancient Greece when a minority of privileged 'citizens' participated in public life (as every adult man in Athens was entitled to contribute to the ruling of the city) or to the French Revolution of 1789 when the regime was toppled in the cause of returning power to the people. However, it is probably most helpful for the purposes of this chapter to refer to the work of Marshall whose seminal work on citizenship has informed much of the contemporary debate surrounding citizenship in the United Kingdom. Marshall (1964) described citizenship by dividing it into three elements, involving access to various rights and powers, the development of which can be viewed historically. These three elements are civil rights, political rights and social rights.

Civil rights

Civil rights concern the rights necessary for individual freedom, for example, for freedom of speech, freedom of religion and the right to justice. These were essentially eighteenth century developments.

Political rights

Political rights concern the right to participate in the exercise of political power, either by exercising a right to vote or standing for political office. Such rights were gained during the extension of the franchise which began in the 19th century.

Social rights

Social rights concern:

> *the whole range from the right to a modicum of economic welfare and security to the right to share to the full in the social heritage and to live the life of a civilized being according to the standards prevailing in the society.*

(Marshall, 1964, p72)

Social rights are twentieth century developments. Marshall stated (see the above quotation) that there was no universal principle determining what the rights and duties of citizenship should be. When he says 'according to the standards prevailing in the society', it would appear that a relative concept is being described. However, he believed that an image of ideal citizenship was being created in societies in which citizenship was developing, and that progression towards this ideal state involved moving towards greater equality between members of society:

Citizenship is a status bestowed on those who are full members of a community. All who possess the status are equal with respect to the rights and duties with which the status is endowed

(Marshall, 1964,p84)

Marshall's 'citizenship and social class' essay was first presented as a lecture in 1949. He was writing, therefore, at an important time in the history of welfare in Britain, as it was during this period that the welfare state was being established. During the Second World War a committee chaired by Sir William Beveridge produced the famous Beveridge Report on Social Insurance and Allied Services, published in 1942. Beveridge stated that there were five giants that needed to be conquered in order to achieve post-war reconstruction. These five were want, disease, ignorance, squalor and idleness. The post-war system was to be based on the principle of universal rights and a minimum income.

Prior to the establishment of the welfare state, social security provisions were largely selective, that is, they provided for certain occupational and income groups and were directed towards the needs of particular individuals. Further, much welfare provision came from the voluntary sector. Following the establishment of the welfare state, services were to be universal, that is, to provide for everyone as a matter of right. For example, the 1945 Family Allowance Act provided weekly cash payments for each child excepting the first; every family in the land was entitled to those payments.

The Beveridge Report aimed to provide for people's needs 'from the cradle to the grave'. The Report's recommendations were put into effect by a series of Acts of Parliament from 1944 to 1948; together they created the modern welfare state in the UK. The developing welfare state assumed more responsibilities for the welfare of the people, for example, widening provision of state education and health care free at the point of delivery. Thane (1982) explains how this change from an emphasis on voluntary action to one on state action is sometimes explained in terms of the growth of citizenship. The social rights addressed by the welfare state would ensure a certain level of material well being that would enable citizens to participate in society.

While there are a range of definitions of the term citizenship, there is agreement on the view that citizenship concerns the relationship between the individual and the state. Oliver and Heater (1994) describe citizenship as follows:

> *The social dimension to citizenship involves the acceptance that the state owes certain services to the citizen as a right in return for the loyalty and services rendered by the citizen. It is part of the reciprocal relationship between the individual and the state which is central to the concept of citizenship* (p20).

This may be viewed in terms of a 'contract' between the citizens and the state. According to this view, citizenship can be viewed as involving certain rights and duties. Duties often take the form of national insurance contributions, obeying the law, undertaking jury service, or attending compulsory education. Other civic duties include the general obligation to be a good citizen having regard for one's fellow citizens and promoting the welfare of the community.

So far, citizenship has been described as a series of rights (often conferring powers) and duties mediated through the relationship between individual and state. Another dimension to the concept of citizenship is offered by Steenbergen (1994) who extends the definition of citizenship to encompass a greater emphasis on the relationship of the citizen with society as a whole, a citizen being one who has a sense of belonging to a community and participates in public life. Oliver and Heater (1994) consider whether the introduction of the welfare state strengthened an already strong sense of community and made it possible for all individuals to feel that they were fully respected members of society; they suggest that citizenship could be taken for granted. However, Cochrane (1993) argues that even where welfare citizenship was taken for granted, not all citizens were equal.

George (1992) argues that social policies can maintain or change relationships between groups, for example, between rich and poor, between the healthy and those with poor health or disabilities. He also argues that these policies can segregate or integrate, sustain or diminish discrimination, and increase or decrease inequalities in resources. Titmuss's (1970) powerful example of blood donation can be used to illustrate this argument. Titmuss examined the extent to which certain aspects of social policy encourage or discourage, foster or destroy the expression of altruism by individuals and regard for the needs of others. Blood donation was investigated in various countries including Great Britain and the United States of America. Similarities and differences were found in the systems used. On the one hand, Titmuss identified the paid blood donor in the USA. Titmuss argued that as the selling of blood took place as a market transaction information concerning the quality of the blood might be withheld from the buyer, resulting in possible harm to the recipient. On the other hand, the voluntary donor in Great Britain gave his or her blood freely to an unnamed stranger. At the time of writing the lowest incidence of post-transfusion hepatitis was seen where commercially supplied blood was avoided. Titmuss argued that the British blood transfusion service could be understood only within the context of the National Health Service, universal and free at the point of delivery, not socially divisive, and which allows people to give or not to give blood for unseen strangers. This leads Titmuss to suggest that the way society structures its social institutions, particularly health and welfare, can encourage or discourage such altruism.

Citizenship in the 1990s

Policies of the 20th century are much more egalitarian than were preceding policies. However, even in 1982, Thane was asking if citizenship had been extended equally to all. From 1945 to the early 1970s the main political parties seemed to accept a broad consensus on politics that served to extend citizens' rights (Faulks, 1994). Goals of welfare provision were broadly accepted by both the Labour and Conservative parties. Why, then, has citizenship become popular again in the 1990s? Oliver and Heater (1994) argue that it is felt by many that the emphasis on individualism in the 1980s discouraged a sense of community responsibility. While the welfare state of the 1940s aimed for a minimum standard of living, and for most people this has been achieved, in the 1990s basic needs are not being met for a significant minority, for example, homeless people and poor people (IPPR, 1993). Brindle (1996) cites evidence from the Child Poverty Action Group that shows that whereas in 1979 14% of the British population was living on or below the level of income support benefit, in 1992 the corresponding figure was 24%. Thus it can be argued that there has been an erosion of some people's social rights. There has been a move away from a universal provision of welfare services to more selective provision, essentially providing for individuals who are deemed to be most needy. This has been achieved through a significant shift towards the 'targeting' of benefits through meanstesting (Dean, 1994). Non-contributory benefits like child benefit have not kept up with inflation and old age pensions have been linked to prices, rather than earnings, at a time when earnings were rising faster than prices. Without doubt, since 1979, there have been moves to reduce the number of people who are dependent on the state for services and support, and to increase the role of the voluntary and private sectors. It has also been a belief of the succession of Conservative governments since 1979 that a reduced role for the state in the provision of welfare services is desirable in order to secure freedom for individual citizens. Such changes in policy have lead Faulks (1994) to assert that the philosophy introduced by Mrs Thatcher amounted to a substantial restatement of the relationship between the government and its citizens.

Social rights have also been placed on the political agenda as a result of the European Union's Social Charter. This is a document which aimed to ensure improved living and working conditions, collective bargaining, vocational training, worker participation in management. The British government did not assent to this document, nor with the subsequent Social Chapter attached to the Maastricht Treaty of European Union. An opt-out of the Social Chapter was secured by the British government. However, while these are important documents, they are essentially addressing rights for workers and not far-reaching citizenship issues (Hantrais, 1995; Twine, 1994).

As well as issues relating to social rights, there have been concerns in the area of civil and political rights which have also inspired the current interest in citizenship. Examples include miscarriages of justice and concern that the party in power, through a powerful prime minister, rather than the electorate, may have been controlling parliament. Dissatisfaction has been expressed with the first-past-the-post electoral system which, some argue, does not fairly reflect voters' opinions.

Against the background of such concerns, calls have been made for constitutional changes, for example, a written constitution (a formal statement of how the British state should be run) and a Bill of Rights (a written statement of individual rights guaranteed by law). Britain has neither, and is the only country in the European Union without a written constitution.

The organisation called Charter 88 has campaigned for electoral and constitutional reform, calling for a new constitutional settlement which would:

> *Enshrine, by means of a Bill of Rights, such civil liberties as the right to peaceful assembly, to freedom of association, to freedom of discrimination ... Create a fair electoral system of proportional representation. Draw up a written constitution, anchored in the idea of universal citizenship, that incorporates these reforms.*

(Andrews, 1991 p 209–10)

Steenbergen (1994) argues that over the past five years, more and more social problems and questions have been formulated in terms of citizenship and civic society. Essentially, the response from the political right has emphasised the duties citizens owe and the obligations of people to engage in 'active citizenship'; while the political left has emphasised citizens' entitlements and notions of 'communitarian citizenship' and more egalitarian policies.

Active citizenship

Oliver and Heater (1994) state that, for many reasons, citizenship in Britain has come to be regarded as problematic, and the promotion of 'good citizenship' is seen as a possible solution to many of the ills of society. The idea of good citizenship in terms of 'active citizenship' has been promoted since the late 1980s. Hurd (1988) describes three traditions that are central to conservative philosophy and that underpin social policy: these are diffusion of power, civic obligation and voluntary service. Citizenship is seen in terms of economic independence from the state. Active citizenship involves activities such as self-help, local community voluntary work and involvement in crime prevention. It is believed that the government cannot legislate for neighbourliness, neither can it create good citizens; it can merely create the conditions in which good citizens can emerge and flourish.

Citizen's Charter

Another response to the increased interest in the concept of citizenship has been the creation of the Citizen's Charter. The Conservative party's Citizen's Charter is essentially about public services and emphasizes the individual's right to good service, information and channels of complaint. As such, the Charter aims to empower individual consumers of services. The background to the Charter can be located in the increasing demand for services. Convinced that sufficient government money was being spent on public services, the government sought other ways of improving services, and perhaps more importantly, improving customer satisfaction by deflecting dissatisfaction away from government and towards the staff running the public services (Oliver, 1993).

The initial Citizen's Charter has been supplemented by particular charters, for example the Patients' Charter and the Parents' Charter. The Patient's Charter was introduced in 1991 in order to inform people of their rights and the standards of service they could expect to receive from the National Health Service. Rights include the right to receive care on the basis of clinical need, not on ability to pay, lifestyle or any other criteria, as well as respect for privacy, dignity and religious and cultural beliefs. Questions can be raised about the efficacy of the Patient's Charter, for example, Richardson et al (1994) describe a research project investigating respondents' views, experiences and knowledge of health services. Respondents were contacted via classes teaching English for Speakers of Other Languages, English as a Foreign Language and through community groups. Findings revealed that 84.4% (65) of the respondents either had not heard of the Patient's Charter or did not reply to the respective question.

Yet citizenship is more than being aware of rights in relation to public services. It is about a sense of community; about citizens acting in harmony. The Citizens' Charter says nothing about the relationship between the individual and the state and as such may be viewed as de-politicising. For example, the rights expressed in the Patient's Charter are described as 'not legal rights but major and specific standards which the Government looks to the NHS to achieve, as circumstances and resources allow'.

Second class citizens

A significant feature of citizenship is egalitarianism. In practice, however, many groups feel that they are 'second-class citizens' (Oliver and Heater, 1994). Oliver and Heater (1994) state that the largest of these second-class citizen groups is women, while others include cultural, ethnic or religious minority groups and homosexuals. Not to be forgotten are people suffering extreme poverty. This view is supported by Faulks (1994) who argues that the study of citizenship relates to issues of gender, race, poverty and class by asking who is included or excluded from citizenship rights. People with disabilities might also be added to this group.

It is necessary then to examine some of these groups in relation to their exclusion or inclusion in society. Ungerson (1993) discusses how, while citizenship is linked with rights and is located in the public domain, caring occurs in the private and domestic domain, where it is difficult to enforce rights. Many women, as a result of their long-term caring roles, may find themselves excluded from society because of poverty in later life. Ginn and Arber (1992) show how there are wide differences among elderly people in their access to resources that promote independence and enable full participation in society. They show how inequality in material, health and caring resources in later life is structured by gender as well as class, with elderly women disadvantaged in all three. Women's relative lack of participation in paid work has implications for financial security in later life through lower income from occupational and private pensions. Women live longer than men but have worse health. Also, in later life, women are more likely to be living alone, dependent on informal care or state services. A social right of citizenship must recognise the contribution to society of the unpaid labour of women (Twine, 1994).

Minority ethnic groups face discrimination at many levels in society. Just to take the example of employment, or rather unemployment, in the period 1989–91, the male unemployment rate for black people and other minority ethnic groups was 13%, nearly double the rate for white people which stood at 7%. Similarly the corresponding unemployment rates for women were 12% for black and minority ethnic group women and 7% for white women (Oppenheim, 1993). Oppenheim further states that, during the same period, over a quarter (29%) of men from black and other minority ethnic groups worked in the distribution, hotels and catering sectors, compared with 16% of white men. (Wages in these sectors are particularly low.)

Unemployment results in considerable financial loss to the people affected and also their families. The risk of unemployment is higher for those in unskilled occupations. Unemployment results in poverty, low self-esteem and social isolation (Benzeval *et al*, 1995). Higher rates of morbidity are experienced by unemployed people as well as raised mortality levels and lower levels of psychological well-being. Twine (1994) reminds us that major problems arise for people and their families if they become unemployed. They become dependent on charity or publicly provided assistance. Thus, unemployment causes dependency. Yet most people do not choose to be unemployed, but are required to be unemployed in the interests of society, for example, due to policies to control inflation, to technological modernisation or to the ebb and flow of markets. They are bearing the costs of other people's progress as the economy changes (Twine, 1994). Unemployment affects the most vulnerable people in society such as unskilled people, disabled people, older people, and people from minority ethnic groups. Issues such as these lead Held (1991) to question whether existing relations between different social classes, or ethnic groups, allow citizenship to become a practical reality.

While Marshall's concept of citizenship may be set in the mid-1900s, the current debate, in the 1990s, takes place in a vastly different society. Beveridge's plan was underpinned by certain assumptions such as the maintenance of full employment. It was also assumed that there was a fixed amount of illness in society and once this was addressed demands on the National Health Service would reduce. Amidst population growth, increase in life expectancy and the increase in technology, it has been difficult to maintain the original ideals. One of the aims of the reformed National Health Service is to be more responsive to the needs of users. Needs-based services in the context of finite resources have resulted in targeting and priority setting. One example is the media report (Macintyre and Hall, 1994) of a 73 year old man with chronic arthritis who allegedly had his regular physiotherapy discontinued as he was over 65 years of age. Fears abound of equitable provision of health care being threatened by fundholding general practitioners and opted out trust hospitals developing 'commercial' principles when competing for contracts in the internal market. The National Health Service, however, was not set up to respond to consumer demands; rather central planning would determine overall priorities in the distribution of resources (Klein, 1992). George and Miller (1994) remind us that governments in all advanced industrial societies are confronted with the increasing public demand for high quality welfare provision.

The Commission on Social Justice was set up in 1992 by the late John Smith, then leader of the Labour Party, 50 years following the Beveridge Report. The task of the Commission was to perform an independent inquiry into social and economic reform in the United Kingdom. The Commission on Social Justice (1994) addresses the five great evils of want, idleness, ignorance, squalor and disease identified by Beveridge in his report. However, the Commission adds a further evil, that of racial discrimination, which, they acknowledge, is a complex problem, interrelated with the larger picture of class and gender inequalities. They also go beyond the issue of race to include discrimination against groups defined by their cultures and religion. Parek (1991) points to the benefits to British society of the presence of people with cultural differences. A wider range of lifestyles is available to all, with different traditions stimulating new ideas. What is needed, according to Parek, is the involvement of minority groups in shaping the future of British society in order to locate and secure their place in it. Thus Parek calls for a politics of citizenship that promotes both the rights of communities with regard to each other, in terms of the recognition and acceptance of cultural diversity, and their obligations in terms of sensitivity to the majority culture.

Citizenship and nationality

At a first glance citizenship indicates a certain kind of exclusivity: someone is a citizen of a country because he/she has certain legal protections and entitlements that do not apply to outsiders (Barry, 1990). Most states have rules about who is born with nationality and how nationality can be acquired (Oliver and Heater, 1994), as it is the state that determines who are citizens. States may utilise the principle of *jus soli*, which relates to the birthplace of any individual, or the principle of *jus sanguinis*, determined by parental nationality and relating to blood. Examples of countries within Europe employing the *jus soli* principle are Belgium, France, Spain and the United Kingdom, while examples of countries employing the *jus sanguinis* principle are Denmark and Germany (Baldwin-Edwards, 1991). Even when the principle of *jus soli* is used, few European countries automatically treat as citizens anyone born within their borders (The Economist, 1991) as other criteria often have to be met. Foreign nationals residing in a another nation state may not enjoy the full range of citizenship rights. This has become particularly important since Article 8 of the Maastricht Treaty of European Union stated that every person holding the nationality of a member state of the European Union shall be a citizen of the European Union. European citizens are entitled to vote in local government and European Parliament elections in the state in which they reside. Further, discrimination is proscribed against citizens of member states on grounds of nationality. Rights and duties of citizenship of the European Union are limited to the nationals of member states and are not available to all individuals regardless of nationality. Many European countries have substantial populations of people who are nationals of non-member states who will not be citizens in the European context. This is important as the World Health Organisation (1992) states that among the possible trends in a future Europe is increased migration both from outside Europe and within.

Another dimension to European citizenship is the freedom of movement that is afforded to citizens of member states, resulting in the potential for many Europeans as well as non-Europeans to live and work in countries other than their countries of birth. Abel-Smith *et al* (1995) state that the most striking observation about the pattern of health and disease in European member states is its diversity. It is important therefore, not to assume homogeneity amongst the population of Europe. People from different European countries have different cultures: Bill Bryson, in his account of his travels around Europe, wrote:

> *I wanted to be puzzled and charmed, to experience the endless, beguiling variety of a continent where you can board a train and an hour later be somewhere where the inhabitants speak a different language, eat different foods, work different hours, live lives that are at once so different and yet so oddly similar.*

(Bryson, 1991 p28)

Reflections on European holidays are likely to support this view.

Citizenship and health

The Institute for Public Policy Research (IPPR) (1993) identified 'the opportunity to enjoy good health' as one of the 'five great opportunities' that should be the basis of social cohesion and economic security. It is identified as a collective as well as an individual responsibility. However, it is widely acknowledged that there are differences in health experiences between various groups in Britain.

Inequalities in health

The starting point for any discussion relating to inequalities in health is often located in the Black Report (Townsend and Davidson, 1988), an influential document that was the outcome of an attempt authorised by government to explain trends in inequalities in health in Britain and to relate these to the policies intended to promote health. The Working Group that produced the Black Report on Inequalities in Health completed its review in 1980, having identified that lower occupational groups, experienced poorer health than people in higher occupational groups. This difference applied at all stages of life.

The Black Report covered the 20 years up to the early 1970s. During this period mortality rates for both men and women aged 35 years and over in occupational classes I and II had declined, while those in classes IV and V showed little change or had deteriorated (Townsend and Davidson, 1988). Such findings were of particular concern as they arose against a background of more than 30 years of a National Health Service committed to equality of access. However, the Working Group argued that social and economic factors, such as income, work, environment, education, housing, transport and lifestyles, all affect health and all favour the better off. A key concept relating to inequalities in health is material deprivation; thus much of the problem lay outside the scope of the National Health Service.

The Working Group had also been charged with identifying policies to promote health and, while they produced 37 recommendations, the major thrust was that more emphasis should be placed on prevention of ill health and the promotion of primary health care, while also improving the material conditions of poorer groups. By the time the Working Group had completed its task there had been a change of government and the recommendations were not well received.

In 1986 the Director General of the Health Education Council commissioned a review of the evidence on inequalities in health which had accumulated since 1980. This review, the Health Divide (Whitehead, 1988), was reported in 1987 and followed a very similar format to that of the Black Report. The evidence confirmed that inequalities in health persisted in the 1980s, demonstrating that most of the major and minor killer diseases affected the poorest occupational classes more than the rich (Whitehead, 1988). Evidence of occupational class differences in mortality applied at every stage of life, from birth through to old age. As well as occupational class, various studies had used other indicators of wealth, such as housing and car ownership. Taking housing as an example, owner-occupation of housing was found to be associated with lower mortality than private tenancy or local authority tenancy.

Unemployed people were also found to have much poorer health than those in work. The Institute for Public Policy Research (1993) stated that unemployed men and women are 30% more likely than the population as a whole to face a chronic long-standing illness or disability.

In the 1990s discussion concerning housing has gone beyond type of accommodation to lack of housing; research performed by CRISIS (Citron *et al*, 1995) found the highest prevalence of tuberculosis ever recorded amongst homeless people in the UK, 200 times the current tuberculosis notification rate in England and Wales.

Explanations for inequalities in health

Various theoretical positions have been offered to explain inequalities in health. Townsend and Davidson's (1988) account of the Black Report (1980) describe artefactual, selectivist, materialist and cultural/behavioural explanations.

Artefactual explanations for inequalities in health involve the use of data that are possibly misleading or inappropriate, rendering the findings of a study invalid. Whitehead (1988) was later to conclude that health inequalities could not be explained by artefact. Smaje (1995) however pointed to the possibility that artefact explanations could apply in studies concerning minority ethnic groups because of lack of adequate data relating to minority ethnic group health.

Selectivist explanations suggest that inequalities in health result from social mobility; healthy people are able to acquire better jobs and so become concentrated in the higher social groups. It is health that determines an individual's social position, according to these explanations. In terms of migrants, Smaje (1995) describes positive selection where healthy and ambitious people may travel seeking to improve their prospects, while negative selection may occur when less healthy people move from communities which may not be able to support them.

Materialist explanations refer to correlations between low socio-economic status and poor health, for example, the effects of being unable to afford a healthy diet, living in unsatisfactory accommodation and the stresses of unemployment. Inequalities in health are found in all modern societies; people who live in disadvantaged circumstances have more illnesses, greater distress, more disability and shorter lives than those who are more affluent (Benzeval *et al*, 1995). Benzeval *et al* (1995) state that in Britain mortality rates at all ages are two to three times higher among disadvantaged social groups than the more affluent. The difference in rate of illness and premature death is wide and increasing and can mean eight years difference in life expectancy. Evidence is cited by Benzeval *et al* (1995) claims that 42000 fewer deaths each year of people aged 16–74 would occur if the death rate for people with manual jobs were the same as for those in non-manual occupations. That poor people are more likely to suffer ill health than the rich has now been acknowledged by the Department of Health (Mihill, 1995). Cultural and behavioural explanations locate the causes of inequalities in health in individual behaviour; in the choices people make, for example choosing to smoke or eat a diet high in fat. It is sometimes suggested that people are guided to choose health-damaging behaviours by their religious or cultural beliefs (Culley and Dyson, 1993). For example, high infant mortality rates have sometimes been attributed to lack of compliance with Western medical approaches to pregnancy and childcare. However, culturalist explanations ignore issues of power, deprivation and racism (Ahmad, 1993), and can result in victim-blaming.

In response to a debate about whether poor people's less favourable health experience resulted from irresponsible behaviour or from their poverty, Le Grand (1987) proposed an explanation in terms of the theory of human capital. Recognition is given to the fact that people make choices under constraints; these constraints often take the form of material limitations. Health may be viewed as a stock of capital that may depreciate over time because of ageing or illness. Individuals can increase the rate of depreciation by pursuing health damaging activities such as eating unhealthy foods or smoking. Alternatively, individuals can engage in activities such as refraining from smoking, eating a health diet and exercising, which may invest in the stock of capital and so slow the depreciation process. Le Grand suggests that a decision regarding health investment or health consumption will be influenced by the perceived benefits of pursuing an activity believed to form an investment in health and the perceived costs of such an activity.

Further, Naidoo and Wills (1994) describe Becker's 'health belief' model, which suggests that an individual's decisions regarding health behaviour are influenced by an evaluation of its benefits weighed against its costs. For example, the cash saving versus the possible irritability and consequent damaged relationships of giving up smoking, or the possible reduced risk of coronary heart disease versus the increased financial cost of pursuing a healthy diet. However, according to Becker's model, further modifying factors are crucial to the decision making process; these include socio-economic variables and psychological variables, that is, factors which may place constraints on the decision making. Thus cultural and materialist explanations interact.

While there is evidence of health damaging behaviour in lower social groups such behaviour cannot be separated from its social context. Benzeval *et al* (1995) state that three times as many people in unskilled occupations smoke compared with those from professional groups, with particularly high rates being found among unemployed people and young adults with children, especially lone parents. Consequently there is a higher prevalence of smoking-related diseases in disadvantaged groups. Behaviours are determined by the social environment in which people live. Thus it can be appreciated that someone with a low income will make his/her choices concerning health behaviour within the constraints of that income level, for example an hourly paid person may lose income by taking time off work to see a doctor. Further, people on low incomes might also be working in less healthy environments thus depleting their health stocks (Le Grand, 1987).

It is now widely recognised that there are differences in health experience between people in different social classes, but there are also differences in health between minority ethnic groups and the white population, and between individual minority ethnic groups. So, in the 1990s, Smaje (1995) adds three further explanations for inequalities in health relating to minority ethnic groups. Genetic explanations may account for differences in health experience by drawing attention to inherited disorders which may affect the quality of life of small numbers of affected people. Examples are sickle cell disorder which affects people of Afro-Caribbean descent and thalassaemia, another inherited blood disorder, which affects people of Mediterranean, Middle Eastern and Asian descent. Also, there is Tay-Sachs disease, which causes progressive brain degeneration and blindness in children and occurs predominantly in the Jewish population (Hunt, 1995). However, inherited diseases account for only a small percentage of the health problems experienced by minority ethnic groups. The effects of migration are also cited by Smaje as possible causes of differences in health experiences, particularly if migration is enforced as in the case of refugees forced to flee their homes in fear of persecution.

Racism is offered as a further explanation. Culley and Dyson (1993) suggest that material factors associated with social class and poor health are compounded by racism, for example in relation to employment or unemployment, or within the health services, failure to provide health information in appropriate languages or even to provide appropriate facilities. For example, Davies *et al* (1993) comment that in Britain service development in relation to haemoglobinopathies has been fragmented. Smaje points out that these categories of explanation are not necessarily mutually exclusive, and offers as an example the apparently high prevalence of schizophrenia in people of Caribbean origin which might be explained by artefactual, materialist and racist theories.

It has already been indicated that poverty can affect people's health. Poverty affects the lives of a fifth of the UK's population and around a quarter of its children (Oppenheim 1993). The second half of 1980s has seen growing income inequality in Britain, and economic inequality is a significant indicator of disadvantage and a determinant of health. It is important, therefore, to consider the socio-economic position of people belonging to minority ethnic groups. Stubbs (1993) states that too often black people are discussed in research as if they do not also occupy classes and genders. Smaje (1995) also supports this view:

People from minority ethnic populations face the dual problems of racism and an increased likelihood of experiencing poverty and disadvantage, both of which may be expected to affect their health. (p9)

However, not all members of minority ethnic groups suffer socioeconomic disadvantage, but their health may still be affected by lack of understanding of cultural needs. Patel (1993) writes concerning care for black elders that the popular image has been that the extended family provides the care. Badger *et al* (1988) described the underuse of community services by elderly black people particularly those of Afro-Caribbean or Asian origin or descent. Their research addressed the needs of physically disabled, frail elderly and elderly mentally infirm people living at home in central Birmingham, and the community health and social services available to them. Only 7% of elderly and disabled patients and clients of community services were black, although in two of the wards studied around 50% lived in households whose head was born in the New Commonwealth or Pakistan. District nurses tended to hold stereotypical views about elderly black people, believing that they lived with caring families. Further, GPs were not referring their black elderly and disabled patients to district nursing services.

Various authors, for example Ahmad (1993), Balarajan and Soni Raleigh (1993) and Smaje (1995), provide excellent coverage of health issues concerning minority ethnic groups; the reader is referred to these knowledgeable texts for detailed accounts. However, it is widely acknowledged that the evidence relating to ethnic health is fragmentary and much of the data relates to place of birth, giving little information concerning the health of second generation members of ethnic groups. However, diseases of minority ethnic populations do not differ fundamentally from those faced by majority populations (Smaje, 1995). For example, coronary heart disease is the single largest cause of death for men and women from several ethnic groups, including the white population.

As far as minority ethnic groups are concerned, little information was available when the Black Report was being produced. Townsend and Davidson (1988) comment on the fact that race had rarely been assessed in official surveys relating to health. Whitehead's (1988) evidence relates mostly to adult immigrants born outside England and Wales, not British born people of minority ethnic group origin. This lack of available data has further been reported by Balarajan and Soni Raleigh (1993) and Smaje (1995). From the limited information available in the 1980s a varied picture emerged. While mortality rates from lung cancer and chronic bronchitis were lower in most minority ethnic groups than those born in the UK, deaths from accidents were higher in all immigrant groups (Whitehead, 1988). Higher mortality rates also existed for people of Caribbean and African origin from hypertension and strokes.

These findings are still supported by Balarajan and Soni Raleigh who addressed issues relating to health and race within the context of the*Health of the Nation* initiative. Their evidence shows that black and minority ethnic groups are at greater risk in respect of most of the key areas identified in the White Paper. For example, mortality from coronary heart disease is higher in people from the Indian subcontinent and the African Commonwealth. Indeed, in 1995 Balarajan reported that coronary heart disease among persons aged under 65 years born in the Indian subcontinent was 55% above the normal rate in England and Wales. Mortality from stroke is higher in people from the Caribbean, the Indian subcontinent and the African Commonwealth. Other evidence shows that Afro-Caribbeans have higher admission rates to psychiatric hospitals. Diagnostic rates for schizophrenia are high in Afro-Caribbeans and are raised also in Asians. Sashidharan and Francis (1993) note the increased incidence of mental hospital admission amongst migrant groups. Stubbs (1993) cites some evidence to suggest that Irish people face particularly high rates of being diagnosed as mentally ill. Balarajan and Soni Raleigh (1993) also state that socio-economic deprivation places black and ethnic minority populations, particularly children, at higher risk of accidents in the home.

Concerning access to health services, Balarajan and Soni Raleigh (1993) describe how evidence relating to inequalities in health and access to health services suggests that social class is an important factor. As such both white and minority ethnic groups in similar social classes may experience similar problems. However, black and minority ethnic groups may also experience racism and language communication difficulties and cultural misunderstandings. The Audit Commission (1993) found that in addition to all the problems faced by patients who speak English, non-English speakers have particular problems over access to services. Confidentiality may be broken when family members, other patients or non-professional staff are used as interpreters. Further, Hine *et al* (1995) report the findings of the Bristol Black and Ethnic Minority Health Survey which reported low levels of participation in exercise, particularly among South Asian women. Barriers to taking exercise, such as the recommended walking and swimming, included fear of racism – several women reported racist remarks while shopping or visiting parks – and language difficulties.

Rights to health care

The idea of rights to welfare has also become linked with the idea of social justice (Plant, 1992). The Commission on Social Justice (1994) describe the values of social justice as:

> *the equal worth of all citizens, their equal right to be able to meet their basic needs, the need to spread opportunities and life chances as widely as possible, and finally the requirement that we reduce and where possible eliminate unjustified inequalities* (p1).

According to Coote (1992) the idea of 'life chances' is closely linked to the idea of individual empowerment as a requirement of citizenship, which, in turn, entails being able to participate in society. This implies that all individuals must have equal access to education, health care and other services necessary to ensure equal chances in life, and also that no one should be subject to unfair discrimination. It follows then that inequalities in health are socially unjust.

The Commission on Social Justice (1994) stated that the right of equal access to health care should be part of a broader vision of social rights. If citizens are to enjoy a 'right to health', the right to health treatment and care must be seen as fundamental. However, this is a difficult area, as there is no legal right to an absolute level of medical care. The Secretary of State for Health has a general duty to maintain a national health service, but this does not entail a legal right to a particular sort of care for any particular individual (Plant, 1992). The United Kingdom is party to international treaties and conventions that seek to guarantee certain rights. Rights relating to health have long been established in international rights documents (Montgomery, 1992). For example, the right to protection of health (Article 11) is enshrined in the European Social Charter of the Council of Europe (drawn up to deal with the social and economic aspect of the United Nations Declaration of Human Rights), to which the United Kingdom is a party (Lewis and Seneviratne, 1992). Plant (1990) argues that 'at the minimum, a just allocation of resources to the individual from the resources of a society dedicated to health is going to require the equal opportunity to acquire such resources, and this is going to mean that each individual's interest in health should be treated with equal concern and respect' (p26–7). Further, Benzeval *et al* (1995) argue that tackling inequalities in health is a fundamental requirement of social justice for all citizens. This is important, as tackling such inequalities transcends the health status of individuals or groups to concern the health of society as a whole, and has implications for cohesion and the stability of society. Twine (1994) argues that social rights are concerned with establishing the material and cultural conditions for social inclusion and participation in order that the 'social self' can develop. But, as well as the social self, Ginsburg (1992) argues that extending social rights promotes social solidarity. In turn, Bradshaw (1994) argues that social cohesion and a sense of solidarity are important determinants of health status.

> *Individuals are citizens when they practice civic virtue and good citizenship, enjoy but do not exploit their civil and political rights, contribute to and receive social and economic benefits, do not allow any sense of national identity to justify discrimination or stereotyping of others, experience senses of non-exclusive multiple citizenship, and by their example, teach citizenship to others.*

(Oliver and Heater, 1994, p8)

Health care professionals cannot always do much about poverty but are in a strong position to guard against any discriminatory practice in health care and can place individual empowerment within a caring context. Rodwell (1996) defines empowerment as:

a helping process whereby groups or individuals are enabled to change a situation, given skills, resources, opportunities and authority to do so. It is a partnership which respects and values self and others — aiming to develop a positive belief in self and future. (p309)

Opportunities also exist for purchasers of health care to assess the health needs of the local population and to see that these needs are met. Leathard (1994) has further stressed that the rise of the concept of 'user' of services has posed a challenge to the established values and practices of health and welfare professionals. This challenge may force such professionals to work together to mutual benefit as alliances of health and welfare professionals generate a wider variety of solutions to the problems which arise. Leathard also states that a key challenge for inter-professional work is discrimination and equal opportunities. Given the pluralistic nature of society in the 1990s this has never been a greater challenge.

References

Abel-Smith B, Figueras J, Holland *et al* (1995) *Choices in Health Policy. An Agenda for the European Union.* Dartmouth, Aldershot

Ahmad WIU (ed.) (1993) *'Race' and Health in Contemporary Britain.* Open University Press, Buckingham

Alibhai-Brown Y (1994) Strangers, citizens and the siege mentality. *The European.* 13.4.94 p18

Andrews G (ed.) (1991) *Citizenship.* Lawrence Wishart Ltd, London

Audit Commission (1993) *What seems to be the matter: communication between hospitals and patients.* HMSO, London

Badger F, Cameron E, Evers H *et al* (1988) Put race on the agenda. *Health Service Journal.* **98**(5129):1426–7

Balarajan R (1995) Ethnicity and variations in the nation's health. *Health Trends,* **27**(4):114–9

Balarajan R, Soni Raleigh V (1993) *Ethnicity and Health. A Guide for the NHS.* Department of Health, London

Baldwin-Edwards M (1991) The socio-political rights of migrants in the European Community. In: Room G, ed. *Towards a European Welfare State?* SAUS Publications, Bristol

Barry N (1990) Markets, citizenship and the welfare state: some critical reflections. In: Olant R, Barry N *Citizenship and rights in Thatcher's Britain: Two Views.* IEA Health and Welfare Unit, London

Benzeval M, Judge K, Whitehead M (eds.) (1995) *Tackling Inequalities in Health. An Agenda for action.* King's Fund, London

Beveridge W (1942) *Social Insurance and Allied Services,* Cmd 6404, HMSO, London

Bradshaw J (1994) The conceptualization and measurement of need. A social policy perspective. In: Popay G, Williams G, eds. *Researching the People's Health.* Routledge, London

Brindle D (1996) Welfare groups deny 'end of poverty'. *The Guardian.* 17th April, 1996 p7

Bryson B (1991) *Neither here nor there. Travels in Europe.* Secker and Walburg, London

Citron KM, Southern A, Dixon (1995) *Out of the shadow.* CRISIS, London

Commission on Social Justice/Institute for Public Policy Research (1994) *Social Justice. Strategies for National Renewal. The Report of the Commission on Social Justice.* Vintage, London

Cochrane A (1993) Looking for a European welfare state. In: Cochrane A, Clarke J, eds. *Comparing Welfare States. Britain in International Context.* Sage, London

Coote A (ed.) (1992) *The welfare of citizens. Developing new social rights.* IPPR/Rivers Oram Press, London

Culley L, Dyson S (1993) 'Race', Inequality and health. *Sociology Review.* **3**(1): 24–7

Davies SC, ModellB, Wonke B (1993) The haemoglobinopathies: impact upon black and ethnic minority people. In: Hopkins A, Bahl V, eds. *Access to health care for people from black and ethnic minorities.* Royal College of Physicians, London

Dean H (1994) Social security: the cost of persistent poverty. In: George V, Miller S, eds. *Social policy towards 2000. Squaring the Welfare Circle.* Routledge, London

Faulks K (1994) What has happened to citizenship? *Sociology Review,* **4**(2): 2–5

George P (1992) Social policy perspectives. In: Robinson K, Vaughan B, eds. *Knowledge for Nursing Practice.* Butterworth-Heinemann, Oxford

George V, Miller S (1994) Squaring the welfare circle. In: George V, Miller S, eds. *Social policy towards 2000. Squaring the Welfare Circle.* Routledge, London

Ginn J, Arber S (1992) Gender and resources in later life. *Sociology Review.* 2(2):6–10

Ginsburg N (1992) *Divisions of Welfare. A Critical Introduction to Comparative Social Policy.* Sage, London

Hantrais L (1995) *Social Policy in the European Union.* Macmillan, Basingstoke

Held D (1991) Between state and civil society: citizenship. In Andrews G, ed. *Citizenship.* Lawrence & Wishart, London

Higgins R (1993) Citizenship and user-involvement in health provision. *Sen Nurs,* 13(4): 14–6

HineC, Fenton S, Hughes AO, *et al* (1995) Coronary heart disease and physical activity in South Asian women: local context and challenges. *Health Educ J,* **54:** 431–43

Hunt S (1995) The 'race' and health inequalities debate. *Sociology Review.* 5(1): 28–32

Hurd D (1988) Citizenship in the Tory democracy. *New Statesman.* **115**(2979): 14

Institute for Public Policy Research (1993) *The Justice Gap.* IPPR, London

Klein R (1992) Strengths and frailties of a 1942 citizen's charter. Guardian. 4th March, 1992 p23

Leathard A (ed.) (1994) *Going inter-professional. Working together for health and welfare.* Routledge, London

Le Grand J (1987) Health and wealth. *New Society.* 16.1.87. p9–11

Lewis N, Seneviratne M (1992) A social charter for Britain. In: Coote A, ed. *The welfare of citizens. Developing new social rights.* Rivers Oram Press, London

Macintyre D, Hall C (1994) Commons fury over NHS 'bar' on the elderly. *The Independent* 15-4-94

Marshall TH (1964) Citizenship and social class. In: Marshall TH *Class, Citizenship and Social Development.* Doubleday, New York

Martin I (1996) £1m plan to turn neighbours from hell into model citizens. Sunday Times. 4.2.96. p6

Mihill C (1995) Poor suffer more illness than rich. *Guardian.* 24.10.95.

Montgomery J (1992) Rights to health and healthcare. In: Coote A, ed. *The welfare of citizens. Developing new social rights.* IPPR/Rivers Oram Press, London

Naidoo J, Wills J (1994) *Health Promotion. Foundations for Practice.* Bailliere Tindall, London

Oliver D (1993) Citizenship in the 1990s. *Politics Review,* 3(1): 25–8

Oliver D, Heater D (1994) *The Foundations of Citizenship.* Harvester Wheatsheaf, London

Oppenheim C (1993) *Poverty. The Facts.* CPAG, London

Parek B (1991) British citizenship and cultural difference. In: Andrews G, ed. *Citizenship.* Lawrence & Wishart, London

Patel N (1993) Healthy margins: black elders' care - models, policies and prospects. In: Ahmad WIU, ed. *'Race' and Health in Contemporary Britain.* Open University Press, Buckingham

Parston G (1996) The citizens are always right. *Guardian Society.* 27.3.96. p7

Plant R, Barry N (1990) *Citizenship and Rights in Thatcher's Britain: Two Views.* IEA Health and Welfare Unit, London

Plant R (1990) Citizenship and rights. In: Plant R, Barry N, *Citizenship and Rights in Thatcher's Britain: Two Views.* IEA Health and Welfare Unit, London

Plant R (1992) Citizenship, rights and welfare In: Coote A, ed. *The Welfare of Citizens. Developing new social rights.* IPPR/Rivers Oram Press, London

Richardson J, Leisten R, Calviou A (1994) Lost for words. *Nurs Times,* **90**(13): 31–3

Rodwell CM (1996) An analysis of the concept of empowerment. *J Adv Nurs.* **23:** 305–13

Sashidharan SP, Francis E (1993) Epidemiology, ethnicity and schizophrenia. In: Ahmad WIU, ed. *'Race' and Health in Contemporary Britain.* Open University Press, Buckingham

Smaje C (1995) *Health, 'Race' and Ethnicity. Making sense of the Evidence.* King's Fund Institute, London

Stubbs P (1993) 'Ethnically sensitive' or 'anti-racist'? Models for health research and service delivery. In Ahmad WIU (ed.) *'Race' and Health in Contemporary Britain.* Open University Press, Buckingham

Thane P (1982) *The Foundations of the Welfare State.* Longman, London

The Economist (1991) What is a European? *The Economist*, 17.8.91. p36-37

The European. (1996) How MEPs would build a house fit for their citizens. *The European*. 21-17.3.96. p11

Titmuss R (1970) *The Gift Relationship*. Allen & Unwin, London

Townsend P, Davidson N (1988) The Black Report. In: Townsend P, Davidson N, and Whitehead M *Inequalities in Health: The Black Report and The Health Divide*. Penguin Books, London

Townsend P, Davidson N, Whitehead M (1988) *Inequalities in Health: The Black Report and The Health Divide*. Penguin Books, London

Twine F (1994) *Citizenship and Social Rights. The Interdependence of Self and Society*. Sage, London

Ungerson C (1993) Caring and citizenship: A complex relationship. In Bornat J, Pereira C Pilgrim D, *et al*, eds. *Community care. A reader*. Macmillan, Basingstoke

van Steenbergen B (ed.) (1994) *The Condition of Citizenship*. Sage, London

Whitehead M (1988) The Health Divide. In: Townsend P, Davidson N, Whitehead M (1988) *Inequalities in Health*. Penguin, London

World Health Organisation (1992) *Targets for health for all. The health policy for Europe. Summary of the updated edition September 1991*. WHO Regional Office for Europe, Copenhagen

3

Old age in Afro-Caribbean and Asian communities in Britain

Mary Tilki

No discussion of transcultural care would be complete without a consideration of older people from minority ethnic groups. The changing age structure of the population draws attention to the relationship between age, class, race and ethnicity. Much can be learned from the experience of Afro- Caribbean and Asian people who came to Britain in the 1950s and 1960s. Such discussions would illuminate the reasons for migration and demonstrate how individuals and groups coped, adjusted to immigration and to being black or Asian in a 'white' society. They would also testify to the experience of discrimination and disadvantage and reveal how at the end of their lives older migrants are adjusting to having ties in this society as well as in their homeland.

Blakemore (1989) suggests that minority ethnic elderly people should not be seen as 'exotic' specimens but should help underline the point that all members of society possess ethnic and racial identity. A focus on older Asian and Afro-Caribbean people can establish general principles about being old by highlighting the significance of cultural values, traditions, identity, belonging and cultural hetero-geneity. It can also raise issues of being a minority within a minority and the effects of unfair treatment in addition to the process of growing old. By focusing upon this section of the population, this chapter will examine discrimination and in particular consider the added impact of ageing on people from minority ethnic groups.

Relative to the white population over retirement age, and as a proportion of all minority ethnic groups, the overall percentage of black and Asian people in Britain is around 5% (OPCS, 1991) However, currently an increase in this percentage is likely to be rapid due to significant numbers in the pre–retirement age band. It is estimated that a four– or fivefold increase will occur before the end of the decade (Blakemore and Boneham, 1994). Although there are problems with statistics due to underenumeration and uncertainty about official age, it is evident that older people from minority ethnic groups are concentrated in metropolitan areas and a few other regions such as Coventry and Leicester (OPCS, 1991).

Table 3.1: Afro-Caribbean and Asian groups by age in Britain

Group	Under 44	45–60/65	Other60/65
	%	%	%
Afro-Caribbean	72	23	6
Indian	80	16	4
Pakistani	88	11	6
Bangladeshi	86	13	2
White	62	16	4

Adapted from OPCS 1991: 25 Table 5.30

Research limitations

Although there is an increasing body of knowledge about old age, it is fair to say that since longevity is a relatively new phenomenon there is much more to be learned. Kohli (1988) argues that ageing has presented a challenge for sociological theory. We are now seeing the emergence of a sociology of ageing, which treats old age as a fundamental aspect of social organisation rather than as an additional and separate variable (Arber and Ginn, 1995; Bury, 1995). However, it is argued that even less is known about ageing in minority ethnic groups, since studies have mainly focused on the responses of younger people to migration and assimilation. Recent work has concentrated on exploring the extent to which older people have assimilated, with many studies recording continued differences even where ethnic and host communities have lived together for generations (Dreidger and Chappell, 1987; Eurag, 1987). Research has of necessity concentrated on patterns of provision and access, with little attention to social relationships between primarily white service providers and black clients, or to the quality of services provided or the type of provision desirable. There has been little attention paid to the experience of growing old, and to that of being old in a place that is not readily identified as home. Although there is evidence of persistent ethnic and racial distinctiveness in settled communities (Little, 1947; Blakemore and Boneham, 1994), there has been a relative absence of longitudinal studies much needed to inform policy and practice.

However, despite research limitations, lessons can be learned from studies in the Asian (Bhachu, 1985; Blakemore, 1982; Boneham, 1989) and Afro-Caribbean (Bhalla and Blakemore, 1981; Barker, 1984; Rowland 1991; Peach, 1991) communities all of which apply to other groups and in some cases to the indigenous older population.

Diversity not homogeneity

Age is an unpredictable guide to social circumstances or personal behaviour and can mask a variety of roles and physiological states (Blakemore, 1989). It is a mistake to assume that those born within a certain decade, or those who migrated within a particular period, share similar characteristics or experiences. Class, race and ethnicity invariably have a stronger influence than age–related variables. Older people are diverse in their lifestyles, levels of satisfaction and access to material resources and come from a range of cultural, ethnic and religious backgrounds. They will have adhered to their home culture and adapted to British culture to varying degrees, and will have had a variety of experiences related to migration and settlement. There will be a range of feelings about 'home', with some still wishing to return to their place of origin and others having decided to stay. Although older people from Afro-Caribbean and Asian minority groups have much in common with each other and the white population, there is little evidence of homogeneity.

Older Afro-Caribbean people

People from the Caribbean have come from a number of different islands and, having little contact with other islands until arriving in Britain, would have identified themselves as Jamaican, or Barbadian, or whatever, rather than as 'West Indian' (Blakemore and Boneham, 1994). They would have grown up in a British colonial system alongside the influences of other colonising powers that shaped each island differently. Like the Irish, the Caribbeans have had a long history of emigration, having to move either to cities or to Britain and the USA to find work (Lowenthal, 1972). The effect on the home community was vast, and left older people and children without the support of the younger migrants and to a subsequent decline in social, educational and employment opportunities for those left behind (Lowenthal, 1972).

Books written about the early experiences of Afro-Caribbean migrants testify to the hope that soon became disillusionment (Little, 1947; Patterson, 1965; Bryan *et al,* 1985). The migrants who came to their 'homeland' or 'mother country' had to deal not only with outright racism but also with a general coldness and reserve from British people (Patterson, 1965). Although considerable numbers worked alongside British people there was no warmth or friendship.

Older Afro-Caribbeans have experienced remarkable stability of living arrangements and locality of residence, but this stability is more a feature of racism in housing than an expression of choice, since they are not necessarily happy with their neighbourhoods (Blakemore and Boneham, 1994). However the degree of identification and rootedness in a particular area may be a positive factor for older people in later life.

Older Asian people

People referred to as 'Asian' came from countries like India, Pakistan and Bangladesh and, like Afro–Caribbeans, have been influenced by British colonialism. Some Indian people will have spent time in second countries such as East Africa or Mauritius. They came from a range of religious backgrounds such as Islam, Hinduism, Sikhism and Christianity. People from places like Gujurat, Punjab and Sylhet were recruited to fill specific gaps in the labour market and therefore settled in different parts of Britain, often with people from their own community. Early migrants to Britain found themselves in a hostile and unwelcoming society (Shaw, 1988). This required them to rely on each other for accommodation, work and welfare. The young and middleaged women who joined the men had little opportunity to meet white neighbours or to learn English. Community studies in the 1980s generally show that Asian families tended to live in households of six or more (Bhalla and Blakemore, 1981). However, patterns of housing provision in some areas precluded this and in some groups, notably East African Asians there was a growing tendency to live in nuclear groupings (Bhachu, 1985).

Although it is true to say that a large proportion of immigrants were employed in semi-skilled and unskilled manual capacities, a number were engaged in skilled, professional and commercial occupations. Some were educated and highly qualified but were not able to find suitable work or licences to practice.

We are here because you were there

Migration to Britain is not a new phenomenon: the 19th century saw large scale migration from Ireland after the Famine; the 20th century saw Jews fleeing persecution in Eastern Europe. Considerable populations of black people and smaller groups of Chinese and Asian 'lascar' seamen settled in port towns like Cardiff and Liverpool (Smaje, 1995). As today, the most significant migrant populations were from Australia, New Zealand, Canada and America. The history of African and Caribbean people in Britain, and especially in London, goes back to the 17th century when as slaves they lived in relatively good conditions but were none the less slaves. By the 20th century their status as domestic slaves became that of servant, and many either ran away or were freed and settled particularly in London. At the same time a number of black people from Africa and the Caribbean began to occupy professional positions, and an increasing body of students formed part of a privileged and transient population (Fraser, 1993). However, the most significant period of migration began with the arrival of almost 500 immigrants on the Empire Windrush in 1948. The buoyant post war economy led to labour shortages which were met by encouraging and actively recruiting migration from the former colonies of the Commonwealth. Although these migrations were numerically smaller than previous groups of Irish or Jews, it was the arrival of significant numbers with different skin colour that ignited colonial ideologies of 'race' (Smaje, 1995).

Push and pull

Throughout the 19th and into the 20th century the colonies continued to make their own contribution to the British economy; their men fought in both Wars while their native economies were systematically underdeveloped. It was this economic deprivation that encouraged people from the Caribbean and Asian subcontinent to respond so readily to the persuasion and propaganda of recruiters in the 1950s and 1960s. The promise of a better life in Britain attracted not only those who had difficulty finding work but also those who were already in skilled and secure employment (Bryan *et al,* 1985). Although it was not appreciated at the time, the hardship experienced back home was to be a good training ground for what was to follow. Much attention has been concentrated on the 'push' factors associated with migration but Peach (1991) argues that the dynamic feature of the 1950s and 1960s migration was the 'pull' of the demand for labour which could not be filled by the indigenous population. This labour supply had declined for a number of reasons and could not meet the post war expansion in the construction and service sector (Ward, 1978). The inflow of immigrants provided a replacement labour force but what was different in this era was the issue of skin colour (Rex and Tomlinson, 1979).

'They're taking our jobs'

Although there was reluctance to employ black workers, in some industries employers had little alternative because indigenous labour was not forthcoming at the prevailing wage and working conditions. The London Brickworks Company in the Bedford area consistently employed a high percentage of West Indian, Asian, Italian and Polish workers because indigenous labour was unwilling to undertake the physically arduous work on day and night shifts, in hot, dusty conditions. The textile industry also had problems recruiting and retaining labour because of seasonal variations in workforce requirements, 19th century buildings and night work. Their disproportionate participation in the unskilled and semi-skilled sectors was in part due to a lack of skill and experience, and for some, language problems. Immigrant workers were concentrated in the non-skilled sector of the job market because they were willing to do the kind of job deserted by the British worker. This contrasts with the popular perception of migrants taking the jobs of the native workforce (Braham, 1984).

A land of milk and honey?

Although women from the West Indies came to join husbands, a good number were recruited specifically as nursing students and ancillary workers to staff the newly developed National Health Service. For many, the posts for which they were recruited did not materialise as they were channelled into cleaning and catering jobs, or auxiliary nursing. The policy of recruiting black nurses to State Enrolled Nurse training rather than State Registered Nurse courses meant that many were to spend long years trying to achieve what they really wanted (Bryan *et al*, 1985).

The discrimination in employment was reflected in housing and general social life. 'No Blacks No dogs No Irish No kids' were common in advertisements for accommodation or services, and the reality to which migrants were recruited owed more to a nightmare than a land of milk and honey.

Men from the Caribbean and Indian subcontinent came first, found jobs and accommodation and, subject to finances, later made arrangements for wives and family to join them. The 1962 Immigration Act restricted rights of entry and meant that those who had been unable to bring families to join them were to be separated them permanently. As economic conditions deteriorated many were unable to sustain the family at home and were forced to return home with ambitions unfulfilled. But because there was no alternative the majority stayed without their partners and children, who were either refused entry or for whom they could not afford the cost of travel (Bryan *et al*, 1985).

Double jeopardy– a word of caution

The term 'double jeopardy' is used to describe the combined effects of age and race (National Urban League, 1964) and 'triple jeopardy' to explain the combined effects of age, race and poverty (Norman, 1985). Different indicators of inequality are used in studies, but they broadly relate to income, life expectancy, social support, self-esteem, life satisfaction and mental well-being (Blakemore and Boneham, 1994). As discussed in *Chapter 2*, the concentration of people from minority ethnic groups in the lower paid sectors of the labour market has implications for health. It also has a major impact on pensions and subsequently income in later life. This is especially important for women who live longer, and may not have participated in the paid labour market, or who have taken time out in part-time employment to bring up a family. The contribution of the migrant to the family back home, and subsequently to the economy of the homeland, is often forgotten. In 1965, 85% of Caribbean women were supporting families back home, in addition to their family in Britain (Bryan *et al,* 1985). The need to support the family at home dug deeply into the pockets of poor migrants and left little money for savings, holidays or consumer durables. The relative lack of income in old age affects many old people, but may cement inequalities where minority ethnic groups are concerned.

Like other older people in industrialised societies, those from minority ethnic groups experience the devaluation of old age. They also bear the additional economic, social and psychological burden of living in a society where equality remains a myth. The focus on double jeopardy has not really considered whether differences between ethnic groups, or between black and white older people, are widening or narrowing. Although it is clear that those from minority groups do suffer disadvantage, there has been little comparative study which takes account of class (Blakemore and Boneham, 1994). It is frequently assumed that the disadvantages of life will be lessened in old age as the differences between groups are levelled out. Blakemore challenges the idea of old age as a 'leveller' that irons out all social, status and economic differences across classes in old age, and asks whether difference is amplified in old age (Blakemore, 1989). Taylor and Ford (1983) recorded that there was more levelling than there was amplification of difference. Although the gaps between social class and gender narrowed only slightly, there was a loss of nearly all resources over time (Taylor and Ford, 1983). However, what was significant was the decline in health, especially in middle class women.

Although there is no consensus, there is some evidence that increasing age narrows some inequalities and modifies the influence of other variables. Further research must be conducted to establish to what extent the combined effects of ageism and racism impact on elderly black people. There is a particular need to examine the subjective experience of ageing in another land, and to explore what well–being, illness and disability mean to older people from minority groups.

Health patterns and problems

The health of older people from Asian and Afro-Caribbean communities is shaped by a variety of economic and social factors and to a lesser extent by cultural forces. Although there is increasing attention to the needs of older people from minority ethnic groups, the research evidence is limited. Research conducted in a biomedical framework does little to illuminate the dimension of culture as shared meanings, understanding and ways of coping with health problems (Kelleher and Islam, 1996). The study of hospital admissions neglects the significant level of illness treated outside hospital. Self reports of health and life satisfaction may reflect the lower expectations of older people from minority ethnic groups rather than better health (Blakemore, 1982). Differences between ethnic groups and the health needs and patterns of illness in the same cultural group in different parts of Britain are not always known (Donaldson, 1986). Studies rarely provide comparisons between people from the British population and those from minority ethnic groups, so it is difficult to interpret whether one group is worse off than the other.

Despite these and other limitations the research available suggests that the health of older people from minority groups is a cause for concern (Blakemore and Boneham, 1994). Lower mortality rates reflect the relative youthfulness of most minority ethnic populations, with the exception of the Irish. They may also relate a selection effect, which Ebrahim refers to as the 'healthy migrant', suggesting that in order to migrate from the Caribbean, Africa and the Indian subcontinent migrants were required to be healthy. However, as the population ages this is less likely to be significant (Ebrahim, 1992). A number of studies have demonstrated significant levels of morbidity and long term disability in Asian, Afro-Caribbean and other ethnic groups. Existing mortality patterns and the ageing of ethnic minority populations suggest a high level of renal and other associated illness (Raleigh *et al,* 1997).

Marked excess mortality from diabetes is evident in men and women from the Indian subcontinent, the Caribbean and African countries (Raleigh *et al,* 1997). The prevalence rates are high in the sixth decade. Diabetes is also a major factor contributing to blindness, renal failure and heart disease. Cultural beliefs about diabetes, diet and body shape can pose additional problems for the management of diabetes in older people from Asian and Afro-Caribbean origins (Pierce and Armstrong, 1996). Lay people's understanding of the causes of diabetes and the importance of diet and insulin differs from that of professionals but, despite this, people have a sophisticated understanding of their condition (Pierce and Armstrong, 1996). In a study of Bangladeshi people the cultural meaning of certain foods, the need to purchase halal food and the requirement to fast at Ramadan were important issues for people with diabetes (Kelleher and Islam, 1996). Although this study was of one specific community, the issues could be similar in other cultural groups; understanding is crucial to effective advice and care.

Hypertension is also excessive in Asian and Afro-Caribbean groups, but with a particularly high mortality rate in Afro-Caribbean women (Raleigh *et al,* 1997). Although some lessons may be learned from studies in the USA, the beliefs and perceptions of people with high blood pressure have received little attention in Britain until recently. A recent study in Lambeth researched Caribbean patients and a matched cohort of white patients being treated by fifteen general practitioners. The Caribbean clients' understanding differed from the formal medical view, but was not very dissimilar from that held by the white people in the study. Both groups identified stress as a related factor and described anxiety and concern when hypertension was diagnosed. The Caribbean group were significantly more likely to see stress as the only cause of high blood pressure, in contrast with the white group who believed the cause was multifactorial (Morgan, 1996). There was also a far greater acceptance of the inevitability of hypertension in the Caribbean cohort. This appeared to reflect the prevalence of hypertension in the community and their familiarity with the problems it caused. This familiarity in some way appeared to reduce its threatening nature despite considerable awareness of the risks. There was an appreciation of the significance of salt in the diet; Caribbean people placed a strong emphasis on the importance of fresh food, as opposed to frozen or tinned. The other important difference was that Caribbean people were much less likely to consider being overweight as a contributory factor. Although both groups were caused stress by the initial diagnosis, Caribbean people did not appear to have perceived themselves as ill, and modified their lifestyle only by avoiding rushing about and getting worked up about things (Morgan, 1996). The beliefs of the Caribbean clients in the study are significant for health promotion and management of hypertension, given the high incidence of stroke and renal disease. Both diabetes and hypertension contribute to high mortality rates and may be amenable to reduction by lifestyle changes and effective treatment regimes that integrate cultural beliefs and practices.

Although Afro-Caribbean people over pensionable age are exposed to a higher risk of stroke, the risk of heart attack is lower than in the white population (Ebrahim,1992; Cruikshank *et al,* 1980). Older Asian people are at higher risk of heart attack by comparison with the whole population of England and Wales (Smaje, 1995). A number of different explanations have been offered, but the diversity of the community and differences in socio-economic status and health behaviour suggest that the link is multi factorial. As in the studies of diabetes and hypertension, Asian people generally had a good understanding of the causes of heart disease, similar to those of white British people (Lambert and Sevak, 1996). Although risk factors like diet, smoking and drinking were cited, there was a strong perception that mental stress was the most significant factor (Lambert and Sevak, 1996).

As would be expected, older people from minority ethnic groups experience hearing impairment, foot and walking problems and dental disorders. Visual impairment is high in the Afro-Caribbean and Asian communities (Bhalla and Blakemore, 1981). While this reflects the high incidence of diabetes, a range of problems other than cataract were also noted. Sight problems in any older person have the potential to limit domestic or social activity and to isolate the person. Problems with osteomalacia varied across different groups and may explain the high incidence of femur fractures in older

Asians, whose diet lacks vitamin D not being fortified by the staples of the British diet. It is not clear why older Afro-Caribbean people appear to have a lower risk of osteomalacia and it may be that over time this will adjust to a similar pattern to the white population. The risk of tuberculosis is higher in people from the Indian subcontinent but may be more a feature of poverty and poor housing than the prevalence in the home country of the migrant (Donovan, 1986).

Studies have shown that between a third and three fifths of older Asian people have difficulty getting outside the house (Blakemore and Boneham, 1994). Although this may well be due to physical incapacity, structural factors are also important. Transport and access to either their own home or shops and facilities may discourage people from going out. Many older people fear crime; this is amplified for older black people who may be subject to racial harassment in addition to the hassle and persistent jibes that other old people are exposed to.

Mental health

Although there has been research into the mental health of people from minority groups there has been limited attention to that of older people. Mental illness in older people is frequently undiagnosed, misdiagnosed or inappropriately treated (Gearing *et al,* 1988). There is no reason to assume that the picture is any better for those from minority groups. Studies of primary care attendance suggest that age and sex standardised rates of mental disorder are low in Caribbean attenders (Smaje, 1995; McCormack and Rosenbaum, 1990).

Community studies have shown a low incidence of psychological symptoms using standard assessment instruments (Williams *et al,* 1993). Both studies pose questions of ethnocentricity in practice or in assessment tools, which fail to detect the differentiated presentation of mental illness in people from minority groups and also in old age. There is also an assumption that the stigma of mental illness in minority ethnic communities prevents uptake of services. There is no evidence that demonstrates that stigma is any greater in one group than another, but what is clear is that there are fears about admission to hospital and a lack of knowledge about the treatments that are available (Blakemore and

Boneham, 1994). Migration is a stressful experience and may well leave lasting scars. The need to survive may protect until other variables intervene. When the family leaves home, ill-health or relocation lead to isolation and depression may occur. There is a need for research that examines ideas of psychological well-being and the experience of being ill, as well as research that pays attention to dementia and depression in specific cultural groups. It is also imperative that the possible buffering effects of social support that traditional and religious beliefs play in the prevention of mental illness in different ethnic communities are explored in order to inform practice and policy initiatives.

Access to services

Studies of access to healthcare services conflict: some suggest low rates of uptake (Blakemore, 1982; Donaldson, 1986; Pilgrim, 1993); others show no difference from that of the indigenous population (Ebrahim *et al*, 1991). Patterns of access to hospitals and general practitioner vary, as does uptake by men and women and people from different groups (Smaje, 1995). Older caribbean people were more likely to have visited hospital in comparison with whites or South Asians; women were the more frequent users (Blakemore, 1982). Gujarati attenders at a GP practice in North London were four times more numerous than an age-matched sample of whites (Ebrahim *et al*, 1991).

The GP Morbidity Survey, standardised for age, demonstrates high rates of consultation among older Caribbean born men and women for endocrine, metabolic, circulatory and ill–defined conditions (McCormick and Rosenbaum, 1990). Caribbean women also consult about neoplasms and skin disorders while men seek help more often with mental health problems. Men and women from the Indian subcontinent also consult about endocrine, nutritional and metabolic disorders as well as a range of digestive, neurological and musculo-skeletal problems. Women are less likely to consult about mental health.

There is some evidence that Asian men experience delay in being referred to regional cardiothoracic centres, are under- diagnosed and have less surgical intervention (Smaje, 1995). Although the impact of this on outcome and mortality is unclear it raises issues of racism in access to services and may be highly significant for the growing numbers of older Asian people in Britain.

Family and social support networks

It is commonly assumed that older people from minority groups have a large and supportive family who are willing and able to care for them. However, a number of older people form Afro-Caribbean and Asian origins have few social contacts or family support. Many older Caribbean people do live within an extensive network of friends and family but significant numbers live alone. Life in the older Caribbean community is relatively individuated and home centred, as despite a network of family and friends older Caribbeans are often scattered (Blakemore, 1994). It is unusual for people from the Caribbean to live in three generation households although they may live in close proximity to the family. Despite the myth of the large family many West Indian men and women are single, have never been married or whose marriage has broken down. Living alone in itself does not signify isolation and many lead full independent lives. Men in particular appear to have active social lives outside the home. However, when very old age and frailty or sickness occur there may be no relative nearby to help. Afro-Caribbean men are more likely to find themselves relatively isolated in later life, while women tend to be in touch with their daughters and grandchildren. Higher rates of illness and fear of crime mean many West Indian women are reluctant to go out but enjoy a home–centred life occupied by cooking, housework, needlework and reading. However, as the population ages women are increasingly likely to be isolated and men in need of support. The place of the church in the lives of older people from the West Indies is crucial. Churches with traditional and modern approaches to Christianity fulfil religious and social roles especially for older women, strengthening psychological and spiritual resources and providing identity in later life (Bhalla and Blakemore, 1981).

Co-residence is common in the Asian community and a large number of older people live with their families in large multi–generation households (Gunaratnam, 1993). This is not just to do with custom but relates strongly to the value of family attachment in the

Asian community (Blakemore, 1994). However, there is also evidence of a surprising degree of isolation in the Asian community despite the family network. Cultural convention, language difficulty and adverse climate cause many to feel incarcerated and abandoned in the home as the family go about their daily business. The status of older people in some Indian societies can be ambivalent and old people are not always afforded the degree of respect one is led to believe they are (Blakemoreand Boneham, 1994). Old people, older women and widows without sons can be particularly undervalued. Boneham (1989) cites considerable distress among older Sikh women who feel oppressed and isolated within the family. Women often enjoy the preparation for weddings and religious festivals but a number are left out of involvement in the arrangements for second generation occasions (Blakemore, 1984). Asian men can feel marginalised, and although engaging in social relationships outside the house, feel left out of the women's domain in the home and involvement with younger people. The dissatisfaction experienced by some elderly Asian men and women reflects the devaluation of old age in western society and racial disadvantage that precludes them from appropriate social facilities. Although most Asian people live with others, a significant proportion live with people who are not close relatives or acquaintances from their home country (Barker, 1984). A number of widows live with in-laws only (Coventry City Council, 1986). This is not to suggest that support can be given only by those with blood ties, but it poses questions about what resources such relationships can provide. It cannot be safely assumed that contact with a number of individuals is sufficient, and it is suggested that the quality of a relationship and in particular having a 'confidante' is more important (Murphy, 1988). Further work must be done on the relationship between gender ethnicity and informal care .

Community care

As mentioned earlier there is growing evidence of low numbers of people from minority groups receiving community services (Bhalla and Blakemore, 1981 and 1983; Donaldson, 1986; Cameron *et al,* 1989; Mirza, 1991). This relates in part to lack of knowledge about services available but also reflects ethnocentricity in service provision. Afro-Caribbean people have minimal language barriers and, often having worked in the public sector, appear more familiar with the services that are available but are reluctant to access home care, meals on wheels and other community services. Older Asians, by contrast, are ill-informed about welfare rights and social services. However, even when aware of provision, some are reluctant to use local day services because of language barriers and the fear of not being welcome. Others either do not feel the need, or are prevented from using services, by illness, disability or lack of transport. It is usually assumed that people from Asian origin prefer to stay with the family, but the provision of culturally specific sheltered housing has proved to be popular with older Asians. Asian men were more likely to express an interest in attending a day service if it could be provided locally but women were much less keen to go (Bhalla and Blakemore, 1981).

Failure to access services does not imply a lack of demand and owes more to the inability or unwillingness of providers and practitioners to provide culturally sensitive care. The experience of minority ethnic communities is one where cultural issues, if considered at all, are inconsistently or unsatisfactorily addressed. Although some attempts have been made to address the needs of children and child-bearing women there has been scant attention to older people from minority groups (Cameron et al, 1989).

Informal care

Community services are frequently not offered when an older person from a minority is discharged from hospital because it is assumed that the family do not need, and may even refuse, help (Cameron et al, 1988; Mirza, 1991). West Indian and Asian nurses confirm the obligation of the extended family to provide help and support to their elders, and perceive older British people to be abandoned by uncaring children (Tilki, 1990).

The obligation to care for older relatives is strong in minority communities; the stigma of using community or institutional services can prevent families from seeking help. The reality of being a family carer in an extended network in Jamaica or the Punjab is a very different experience in British society. There may be a limited network of relatives and friends to share the task in a British city. Housing for most is crowded and the need for women to work outside the home or at piecework within the home reduces the capacity for caring. Despite the willingness and the obligation to care there is widespread evidence of the difficulties of informal care. Although as yet there is limited evidence about minority ethnic groups, it would be foolhardy to imagine that it is unproblematic. It would appear that despite the larger and geographically closer nature of the Asian family, the responsibility for caring still falls on one member, in a manner similar to that of the British but with the added difficulties of gaining access to social services (Mirza, 1991). There is as yet little research that considers the meaning of relationships, beyond the assumption that marital or filial relationships are freely chosen, are based on love and nurture personal growth (Askham, 1995). The expectations of the community, the elder and the carer lead to a sense of obligation which may not be the best foundation for a caring relationship. Conflict between generations can happen in any family, but when it reflects differences in cultural values it poses an added stress for both carer and cared for. It is significant that, although older people have more contact with family and friends, they are more concerned about being abandoned or neglected by their families (Blakemore, 1989; Tilki, 1990).

Belief in the duty of care and the stigma of using outside help pose additional stresses for carers from minority groups. Although there is no published evidence to date, anecdotal accounts of elder abuse in minority communities are emerging. Rather than pathologise the minority ethnic family engaged in care, research is needed, not only to identify the extent, but also to examine the qualitative aspects of informal care.

Myth of return

Asian and Afro-Caribbean people who came to Britain in the 1950s and 1960s came to work, to train and to return at the end of their working life. Many still cherish a wish to return and hold a picture postcard image of home in their hearts. It is probably this dream that has helped them survive the difficulties and disadvantage and diverted their dissatisfaction into the hope of return (Blakemore and Boneham,

1994). However, although many would like to live in another country, not all make plans to return home (Bhalla and Blakemore,1981).

Older West Indian people express more dissatisfaction with their lives in Britain, which may relate to the fact that they never intended to stay (Fenton, 1987). Peach (1991) suggests that return migration to the Caribbean is growing. Blakemore speculates that while the evidence on return is inconclusive, those who do go home appear to have escaped poverty and have social ties and other facilities that make for a successful return (Blakemore and Boneham, 1994). Although the longing to be 'home' is expressed widely as people become older, many must reconcile themselves to losing their dream of return. The intention to return home having achieved upward social mobility or enough money to acquire a higher standard of living is strong, but a lifetime of low income, the desire to remain with children and grandchildren and the death or dispersal of family from the homeland discourage many from returning. There are concerns about the services and family networks available to support them in their homeland in later life. There is also a growing sense of no longer being part of the society that they left because of changes in themselves and the home society. Although a number freely and happily choose to stay, they do not lose their ethnic identity and these needs must be met with sensitivity. Older people must be encouraged to keep in touch with their cultural identity which reflects their birthplace and their life in another place. Reminiscence activities, culturally informed leisure pursuits, local community events and intergenerational projects are just some of the measures which might be adopted.

Different needs or not?

Given the diversity of older people from Asian, Afro-Caribbean and other ethnic minority communities it is neither possible nor desirable to suggest a 'prescription' for services. Assessing cultural needs and planning to meet these needs are crucial and must not be left to chance. The model proposed in *Chapter 7* offers a framework for cultural competence that acknowledges issues of ethnicity and takes account of racism in society and in healthcare practice. However, the issues of ageism must be also recognised and challenged. Ageist ideas that presume disability, dependence and passivity must be resisted. The model that relates primarily to cultural competence is based on principles that can be adapted to promote awareness and knowledge about old age. Specific theory is required to inform the practice of caring for older people and should embody the principles of anti-oppressive practice referred to in other chapters. With adjustment our transcultural model can go some way to challenging ageist barriers that currently influence the care that older people receive.

Many of the services needed by Afro-Caribbean and Asian people do not differ substantively from those of the older population as a whole, but for various reasons are not readily accessible to people from minority ethnic groups. Fear of being unwelcome on the one hand and lack of cultural sensitivity on the other prevent older people from using services and may result in crisis intervention at a later stage. Factors like proximity to the home, family or transport may be more significant than cultural specificity and it may be more practical to use clinic, day or residential services that cater for a range of cultural groups. Although many people from ethnic minority groups enjoy mixed company, some would feel more comfortable with people from their own community. Being with people from their own background can help keep them in touch with their heritage and culture, affirm their identity and ameliorate the pain of never seeing 'home' again.

There will invariably be a need to provide specific services for certain cultural, linguistic or religious groups whose needs can not be easily met within mainstream provision. Providing culturally specific services has the potential to benefit the whole community, not just those from ethnic minorities. Cultural awareness and specific cultural know- ledge can lead to the early detection of problems such as hypertension and the complications of diabetes. Culturally informed health advice could enhance the acceptance of dietary constraints, provide culturally appropriate adaptation strategies and increase adherence to therapeutic regimes, thus reducing the likelihood of medical crises such as stroke and long term problems like blindness. Prevention, early detection and effective treatment frees resources for everybody, not just those from minority groups.

Greater uptake and participation by people from specific cultural groups can lead to the development of expertise with both clients and related health issues. This can mean a reduction in complications, more effective and sensitive treatment and greater client satisfaction. Research is needed to evaluate the effectiveness of specific services but it is not difficult to imagine that regular contact and dialogue with particular client groups and their health problems will lead to increasing expertise. Recognition of such expertise may attract funding for research and development and even for service contracts. This should in time prove to be cost-effective with higher scores in terms of client satisfaction, cost-effectiveness and therefore benefits for the whole community.

Services may be best planned and delivered by collaborative partnerships between the ethnic voluntary sector and statutory bodies. Lessons can be learned from good practice that currently exists within the Asian and Afro-Caribbean, Greek Cypriot and Irish voluntary sector in various parts of Britain. Such initiatives offer models for good practice which are applicable to other communities and client groups. However the scale of the voluntary sector and its very nature of being voluntary needs to be protected and its best practice developed. Resources must be ring-fenced over reasonable timescales to ensure adequate strategic planning, to provide security for users and workers and to attract and retain, or to develop, high calibre staff. Collaboration does not always mean cash funding but could involve payment in kind by way of accommodation, transport, administrative support, training, staff development and professional advice. Dissemination of good practice can promote both the voluntary and statutory sector and provide opportunities for dialogue and debate with ultimate benefits for the whole community.

Needs or rights

Health inequalities are socially unjust; being from an ethnic minority group as well as being old can spell significant injustice. Although it is clear that older people from minority ethnic groups have specific needs, it may be more appropriate to consider, in the first instance, that, like members of the indigenous older population, they have rights as citizens. Having contributed to the fabric of British society for decades, older Asian and Afro-Caribbean people, and those from other ethnic groups, have a right to be able to make informed choices and obtain help and support in accordance with their own cultural beliefs. It is simplistic to assume that all clients have equal access to what is provided. Language facilities, information and approachable staff are crucial in enabling older Asian and Afro-Caribbean people and people from other minority ethnic groups to obtain the welfare benefits and mainstream services they currently do not claim. Older people from ethnic minority communities, particularly women, need skilled advocacy to obtain pensions and benefits, to ensure housing rights and to obtain community services. Some also need help to make a will and a few still need to sort out immigration status.

As can be seen from research in the Asian community more could be done to make older people aware of what is available. Attention to cultural sensitivity and community outreach could greatly encourage uptake, not just in Afro-Caribbean and Asian groups, but also in other ethnic minority groups. *Chapter 8* discusses the concept of empowerment: it is imperative that older people from minority ethnic groups should not be passive recipients of services but should be involved in deciding the types of service which are suitable for their particular group. These may be within regular provision for the whole community, or may be specific to particular cultural groups. As with services for younger people, older users should be actively involved at all stages of provision, not just at the consultation stage.

Services must be planned to afford dignity and choice and enable older people to remain within their usual circumstances if at all possible. Every attempt should be made to maintain contact with the neighbourhood and community to allow opportunities for friendship and companionship. Social clubs, day centres and community groups can offer educational and leisure facilities as well as facilities for advice, health promotion or chiropody. Where families choose to care they must be supported by appropriately skilled and culturally competent workers, and by the provision of day, domiciliary and respite care. Service providers should attempt to recruit and train, or reskill, staff from appropriate minority ethnic communities to deliver cultural sensitivity in whatever role they undertake, whether in culture specific or generic services.

It could be argued that the provision of specific services for Asian or Afro-Caribbean or other minority communities is to favour the minority. It might also be argued that to provide specific services is to engender a new type of apartheid. Such arguments rear their ugly heads in times of economic stringency and frequently cause tension between the indigenous population and between individual ethnic groups as they compete for resources. These ideas are little more than thinly disguised racism and fail to recognise the citizen rights of a group who came here predominantly as subjects of the British Commonwealth. They have, in addition to their Commonwealth status, earned their entitlement in British society by their contribution through employment, direct and indirect taxation and human effort, suffering discrimination and hostility in the process. The provision of culturally sensitive services is a civil right owed to those who have fulfilled their obligations in their working lives and deserve a just and decent life in their twilight years. Rather than taking anything from the community, providing culturally competent care for older people from minority ethnic groups has the capacity to enhance the expertise and skill of those directly involved in care and ensure quality of provision for all older people.

References

Arber S, Ginn J, (eds.) (1995) *Connecting Gender and Ageing: A Sociological Approach*. Open University Press, Buckingham

Askham J, (1994) Marriage relationships of older people. *Reviews in Clinical Gerontology* 4: 261–8

Balarajan R, Raleigh V, (1997) Variation in mortality from diabetes mellitus, hypertension and renal disease in England and Wales by country of birth. *Health Trends* 28(1): 122–8

Barker G (1984) *Black and Asian Older People in Britain*. Age Concern, Mitcham, Surrey

Bhachu P (1985) *Twice Migrants – East African Sikh Settlers in Britain*. Tavistock, London

Bhalla A, Blakemore K (1981) *Elders of Minority Ethnic Groups*. AFFOR (All Faiths for One Race), Birmingham

Blakemore K (1982) Health and illness among the elderly of minority ethnic groups. *Health Trends* 14(3): 68–72

Blakemore K (1989) Does age matter? In: Bytheway B ed. *Becoming and Being Old: Sociological Approaches to Later Life*. Sage, London

Blakemore K, Boneham M (1994) *Age, Race and Ethnicity: A Comparative Approach*. Open University Press, Buckingham

Boneham M (1989) Ageing and Ethnicity in Britain: the case of Sikh elderly women in a Midlands town. *New Community* 15(3):

447–59

Braham P (1984) *Class, Race and Immigration.* Open University Press, Buckingham

Bryan B, Dadzie S, Scafe S (1985) *The Heart of the Race: Black Women's Lives in Britain.* Virago, London

Bury M (1995) Ageing, gender and sociological theory. In: Arber S, Ginn J eds. *Connecting Gender and Ageing: A Sociological Approach.* Open University Press, Buckingham

Cameron E, Badger F, Evers H (1989) District nursing, the disabled and the elderly: who are the black patients? *J Adv Nurs* **14:** 376–82

Coventry City Council (1986) Unpublished data ethnic minorities elders survey. In Blakemore K, Boneham M eds.

Cruickshank JK *et al* (1980) Heart attack, stroke, diabetes and hypertension in West Indians, Asians and Whites in Birmingham England. *Br Med J* **293** 25thOctober 1980 1108

Donaldson LJ (1986) Health and social status of elderly asians: a community survey. *Br Med J* **293**(7): 1079–84

Donovan J (1986) *We Don't Buy Sickness, It Just Comes.* Gower, London

Dreidger I, Chappell N (1987) *Aging and Ethnicity: Towards an Interface.* Butterworth, Toronto

Ebrahim S (1992) Health and ageing within ethnic communities. In: Morgan K ed. *Gerontology : Responding to an Ageing Society.* Jessica Kingsley Publishers, London

Ebrahim S *et al* (1991) Prevalence and severity of morbidity among gujarati asian elders: a controlled comparison. *Family Practice* (1):57–62

EURAG (1987) *The Older Migrant.* European Association for the Elderly, The Hague

Fenton S (1987) *Ageing Minorities: Black People as they Grow Old in Britain.* Commission for Racial Equality, London

Fraser P (1993)Africans and caribbeans in London. In: Merriman N ed. *The Peopling of London* Museum of London

Gearing B, Johnson M, Heller T eds. (1988) Mental Health Problems in Old Age. Open University/John Wiley & Sons, Chichester

Gunaratnam Y (1993) Breaking the silence: asian carers in Britain. In: Bornat J *et al* eds. *Community Care A Reader.* Macmillan, Basingstoke

Haskey J (1991) The ethnic minority populations resident in private households. *Population Trends* Spring 22–35

Kelleher D, Islam S (1996) How should I live? Bangladeshi people and non-insulin dependant diabetes. In: Kelleher D, Hillier S eds. *Researching Cultural Differences in Health.* Routledge, London

Kohli M (1988) Ageing as a challenge for sociological theory. *Ageing and Society* **8**(4):367–94

Lambert H, Sevak L (1996) Is 'cultural difference' a useful concept? perceptions of health and the sources of ill-health among Londoners of south Asian origin. In: Kelleher and Hillier *op cit.*

Little K (1947) *Negroes in Britain.* Kegan Paul, Trench, Trubner and Company, London

Lowenthal D (1972) *West-Indian Studies.* Oxford University Press

McCormick A, Rosenbaum M (1990) *Morbidity Statistics from General Practice.* HMSO, London

Mirza K (1991) Community care for the black community. waiting for guidance. In: Central Council for Education and Training in Social Work, ed. *One Small Step for Social Justice: the Teaching of Anti-Racism in Social Work Diploma Programmes,* London

Morgan M (1996) The meanings of high blood pressure among Afro-Caribbean and White patients. In: Kelleher and Hillier *op cit.*

Murphy E (1988) Prevention of depression and suicide. In: Gearing B *et al Mental Health Problems in Old Age.* John Wiley and Sons, Chichester

National Urban League (1964) *Double Jeopardy; The Older Negro in America Today.* National Urban League, New York

Norman A (1985) *Triple Jeopardy: Growing Old in A Second Homeland.* Centre for Policy on Ageing, London

Office of Population Censuses and Surveys (1991) *Labour Forces Survey 1988 and 1989* HMSO, London

Patterson S (1965) *Dark Strangers – a Study of West-Indians in London.* Penguin, Harmondsworth

Peach C (1991) *The Caribbean in Europe: Contrasting Patterns of Migration and Settlement in Britain, France and the Netherlands.* Research Paper No15. Centre for Research in Ethnic Relations, University of Warwick

Pierce M, Armstrong D (1996) Afro-Caribbean beliefs about diabetes: an exploratory study. In: Kelleher and Hiller *op cit.*

Raleigh V, Kiri V, Balarajan R (1997) Variations in mortality from diabetes mellitus, hypertension and renal disease in England and Wales by country of birth. *Health Trends* **28**(4): 122–8

Rex J, TomlinsonS (1979) *Colonial Immigrants in a British City– A Class Analysis.* Routledge and Kegan Paul, London

Rowland DT (1991) *Pioneers again: Immigrants and Ageing in Australia.* Australian Government Publishing Service, Canberra.

Shaw A (1988) *A Pakistani Community in Britain.* Blackwell, Oxford

Smaje C (1995) *Health Race and Ethnicity: making sense of the Evidence* Kings Fund Institute, London

Taylor R, Ford G, (1983) Inequalities in old age. *Ageing and Society* **3**(2): 183–208

Tilki M (1990) *The Social World of the Care of the Elderly Nurse: A Feminist Approach.* Unpublished MSc Thesis, Middlesex Polytechnic

Ward R (1978) Race relations in Britain. *Br J Sociol* **29**(4)

Williams R , Bhopal R, Hunt K (1993) Health of a Punjabi ethnic minority in glasgow : a comparison with the general population *Journal of Epidemiology and Community Health* **147:** 96–102

4

The health needs of the Greek Cypriot people living in Britain

Irena Papadopoulos

The Greeks and Greek Cypriots living in the United Kingdom have never been the subject of a comprehensive survey of their health and lifestyle. This is not surprising, since the recognition by the government, and by health professionals, of the need to study seriously the health variations of ethnic groups living in the UK is relatively recent. Indeed, it was not until 1992 that the Chief Medical Officer's report *On the State of Public Health 1991*, emphasised that many of the government's policies and service development initiatives could not be achieved unless the health of ethnic minorities was improved.

In general terms, even baseline demographic data about the Greek and Greek Cypriot communities has been lacking; the most authoritative source of demographic information in Britain, the decennial census, did not, up until 1971, include any questions relevant to ethnicity. The 1971 census asked for country of birth and that of the parents. By 1991, the census included a list of eight ethnic groups plus a category for 'any other'. In the 1991 census, people of Greek and Cypriot origin were classified as 'white', since these communities were not thought by the Office of Population Censuses and Surveys (OPCS) to be sufficiently large to warrant separate identification, although the census asked the country of birth of the head of household.

Doctors, nurses and other health professionals, as well as medical sociologists, have failed to investigate the health and healthcare needs of the Greeks and Greek Cypriots living in the UK. Possibly one exception has been that of thalassaemia, an inherited type of anaemia which affects not only Greeks and Greek Cypriots but also many who originate from Mediterranean countries.

The survey

The information included in this chapter is derived from a survey of 490 randomly selected Greeks and Greek Cypriots living in the London Boroughs of Enfield and Haringey which I conducted during 1995. These two boroughs are coterminus with the New River Health Authority, now known as the Enfield and Haringey Health Authority.

These two neighbouring north London boroughs have the highest concentration of Greek Cypriots in the United Kingdom. The 1993 publication *New River Sector Profiles* states that the largest minority ethnic group in New River are the Cypriots (Greek and Turkish) who form 6.8% of the total population in the two boroughs. The 1991 OPCS census showed that in Haringey 11,593 residents reported that their head of household was born in Cyprus. This represents 5.7% of the total population of Haringey (202,204 residents on census night). In Enfield, 7.9% are in households headed by a Cypriot, 20,400 residents out of the 257,411 total population of the borough (Enfield Planning Information, 1993). These figures represent both Greek and Turkish Cypriots and are generally considered to give only a part of the total figure. Indeed, in January 1994, the Environmental Services of the London Borough of Enfield, having adjusted the available census figures, estimated that the Cypriots in Enfield numbered 25,000, or 9.5% of the total population. In the absence of any demographic evidence that gives a breakdown of the ratio of Greek to Turkish Cypriots, the London Borough of Enfield have used as a guide the findings of a school language survey which was carried out in the borough in 1990. This survey found that 63% of school pupils were Greek speaking and 37% Turkish.

The sample

The sampling frame for my survey was drawn from the electoral rolls of the two boroughs. A computer programme that was able to recognise Greek names was used to create a list of 2,735 names of Greek and

Greek Cypriot voters in Haringey and 8,433 names of Greek and Greek Cypriot voters living in Enfield.

A postal questionnaire based on the Newcastle Health and Lifestyle Survey (NHLS,1991; Harrington *et al*, 1993) was sent to the sample shown in *Table 4.1*. As can be seen from the table the number of females in the sample were greater than the males (56.7% and 43.3% respectively). Some of the questions were modified or specifically designed for this survey and were tested in the pilot study which included 30 individuals. In my analysis, I will refer to health data available from the Cypriot government, as I believe that this will supplement the meagre data from this country, and will help us understand the health status of the Greek Cypriots in the UK. This position is based on the evidence that the Greek Cypriot community in the UK maintains a strong sense of ethnic identity that influences their lifestyles in similar ways as it does those who live in Cyprus (Anthias, 1992; Constantinides, 1977)

Table 4.1: The sample of the main study

Borough	Males	Females	Total
Enfield	110	139	249
Haringey	102	139	241
Total	212	278	490

Of the 490 subjects, 151 returned their completed questionnaires. Twenty seven were returned by the post office, presumably because the person to whom the questionnaire was sent no longer lived at the address. Another eight were returned with a note stating that the questionnaire was too personal or too long. For various reasons (mainly due to lack of funds as the study was self-funded), reminder letters were not sent to those who failed to returned their questionnaires. Taking into account the returned but uncompleted questionnaires, the response rate was 33.2%. Although it has been hoped that the response rate would be higher, considering the length of the questionnaire and the lack of follow up, this was not totally unexpected.

The questionnaire

The questionnaire consisted of a total of 88 questions (361 variables) which covered the following 12 areas:

1. about yourself

2. about your health

3. food

4. alcohol

5. activity at work and leisure

6. smoking

7. stress in your life

8. about your home, family and social life

9. about your health and your doctor

10. your views about health and illness

11. finding out about health issues

12. your views

Each questionnaire (which was in English only) was accompanied by a letter in English and a letter in Greek, giving information about the study, emphasising the confidential nature of the information given and also asking those who needed help with the completion of the questionnaire to contact me.

Section 1: Characteristics of respondents

Respondents' characteristics are summarised below.

Table 4.2: Summary of demographic characteristics
(*all percentages were rounded*)

Age range:		18–82years	
Marital status:	%	**Household size:**	%
Married	52	No children	61
Single	29	1–2 children	31
Divorced/Separated	7	3+ children	8
Widowed	7		
Cohabiting	5		
Education:		**Employment:**	
Up to secondary	49	Working	47
education	26	Economically active	33
Further education	26	Retired & other	12
Higher education		Unemployed	8
Generation:		**Personal income**	
First generation	56	**range:**	
Second generation	35	Up to £4000	40
Third generation & other	9	£4001–£8000	26
		£8000+	25
		10% did not respond	
House tenure:			
House mortgaged	48		
House owned outright	36		
Renting	16		

Discussion of findings

The report by the STORKEY (1994) *London's Ethnic Minorities: One City Many Communities. An analysis of the 1991 Census results,* states that there were 50,684 people living in London but born in Cyprus. As discussed earlier in this chapter, over 31,000 of them live in Enfield and Haringey. Naturally, Cypriots are both Greek and Turkish and the OPCS statistics do not differentiate, but, considering the demography of Cyprus and the patterns of migration, Anthias (1988) estimates that approximately a quarter are Turkish and the remainder Greek. These figures are grossly underestimated as they exclude households headed by Cypriots born in the UK. It is therefore fair to say that the needs of this large community group must be identified and understood both by health care providers and by those who commission and purchase health services.

The findings of this study indicate that more than half of the respondents are first generation Greek Cypriots. If we consider that just over 20% of the sample are 55 years or over, the relevance of culture and health behaviours becomes obvious. Constantinides (1977) wrote that the interesting point about Greek Cypriots is their potential invisibility within the British majority population. Yet, in spite of this, those who have written about the Greek Cypriots in Britain (George and Millerson, 1967; Oakley, 1970 and 1987; Constantinides, 1977; Anthias, 1992) have commented upon their strong sense of ethnic identity.

Marriage is an important institution within the Greek Cypriot community. Constantinides (1977) found that even second generation Greek Cypriots wished and expected to marry within the community. Once married, it is exceedingly difficult to divorce as the Greek Orthodox Church recognises very few ground for divorce, although recent anecdotal evidence both from Cyprus and the London Greek and Greek Cypriot community seems to indicate an increase in divorce rates, which may reflect an adjustment to social realities by of the church. Cohabiting is generally disapproved of by parents and friends and when it happens those concerned do not freely admit to it. Paschalis (1986) reported, in a study about the position of women conducted in Cyprus in 1978, that 76% of the respondents were definitely against cohabiting, and 83% believed that only in marriage should sexual relations be consummated, thus considering marriage as the only framework of a permanent bond. The findings of my study show a small number of people (5%) who are cohabiting.

The results of my study reveal that Greek Cypriot families are small and similar in size to those of the indigenous population, with the majority of families having 0–2 children. Bearing in mind that there is an over-representation of women in the sample of my study, it is not surprising to find that almost 25% of the respondents described their work status as 'looking after the home and the family'. This finding indicates that these activities remain the woman's domain. It is however likely that many of these women work very hard from home sewing clothes for low wages and outside the employment regulations.This means that they are not legally employed and therefore have no employment rights. Anthias (1992) reported that Greek Cypriot men still expect their wives to be solely responsible for child care and domestic labour even when they work full time. For many women this inequality within the marriage causes enormous stress which sometimes leads to marital difficulties and even physical and mental illness.

Education is also highly valued amongst the Greek Cypriot community. The findings of this study confirm Anthias' (1992) assertion that educational achievement is a dominant value for Greek Cypriots and may be regarded as an important element of class and ethnic adaptation. She reminds us that the Cyprus educational statistics show that more than half of those who complete their secondary education go on to higher education. There are clear parallels between the trends in Cyprus and the UK. As already mentioned above, Greek Cypriots retain a strong sense of ethnic identity. This is both manifested and maintained through regular holidays in Cyprus, through a continued interest about the social, political and economic situation in Cyprus and regular update of these through Greek newspapers, Greek radio and more recently through the reception of Greek television (from Cyprus and Greece) via satellite or cable. My findings show that a high proportion of the Greek Cypriot population are well educated: something that needs to be noted by health providers and purchasers when planning health promotion campaigns or when dealing with them as clients in general.

Home ownership in Cyprus is extremely high; families expect to help substantially towards the purchase of a home, as a wedding gift , mainly for daughters. Owning one's home is considered the foundation of the nuclear family. This attitude is very much evident within the Greek Cypriot community in the UK. It is not surprising therefore that almost 85% of the respondents either own outright or are buying their homes. (Home ownership in the New River Health Authority catchment area by the general public is reported to be in the region of 60%.) To achieve this, many families make enormous sacrifices. The findings about employment and income indicate that the majority of the respondents have low incomes. A large proportion of their income goes towards mortgage repayments; this must have negative consequences on other activities such as leisure, and on the levels of stress experienced by the respondents.

Section 2: Respondents' health status

Physical characteristics

Respondents were asked to record their height and weight. Body Mass Index (BMI) gives a measure of the relationship between weight and height [BMI = weight (kg) / height^2 (m)]. BMI figures were calculated for all those who reported their height and weight. *Figure 4.1* illustrates the proportion of men and women in each BMI category. This shows that very few men or women in the sample were underweight (approximately 6%). The largest proportion of both men and women fell into the 'healthy' category (59% of men and 45% of women). Thirty per cent of the men and 31% of the women were found to be overweight. Women had a greater tendency to be obese (18% versus 6%). BMI also varied with age as the boxplot in *Figure 4.2* shows; as age increases so too does BMI for women although this is not the case for men.

Figure 4.1: Body Mass Index by gender

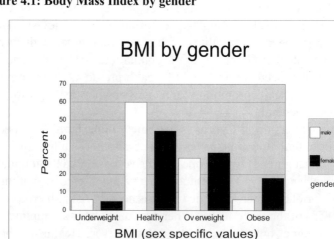

Figure 4.2: Body Mass Index by age and gender

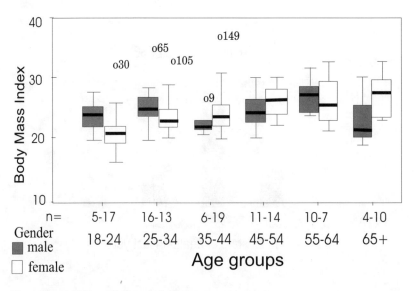

Perceived health and fitness status

Respondents were asked a series of questions about their, and their family's, health. When asked to rate their usual state of health over the past twelve months, a quarter (25%) rated themselves as having been 'very healthy', over half (57%) as 'reasonably healthy', 15% as 'not very healthy', and 3% as 'definitely ill or in poor health'. There were, however, some gender differences as *Figure 4.3* illustrates, and differences between age groups. Nobody in the 18–34 age group described themselves as 'ill or in poor health' and they described themselves as 'very healthy'more often than the middle or older age groups (49% versus 11% and 6% respectively). Most people (57%) described their health as 'reasonable' and the middle age group was more likely to say this than the others.

Figure 4.3: Perceived Health Status by Sex

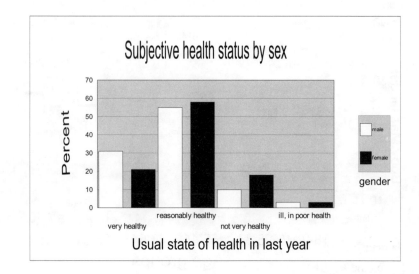

Respondents were asked to rate their present physical fitness for their age using a five point scale. Fifteen subjects (10.1%) rated their fitness as 'very good', thirty seven (24.8%) as 'good', seventy three (49%) as 'reasonable', twenty (13.4%) as 'poor' and four (2.7%) as 'very poor'. Therefore, 83.9% of the respondents considered themselves to be reasonably fit for their age, which is consistent with their perception of their state of health reported above.

Figure 4.4 indicates the fitness levels as they relate to age while *Figure 4.5* relates to fitness and gender.

Figure 4.4: Perceived fitness level by age

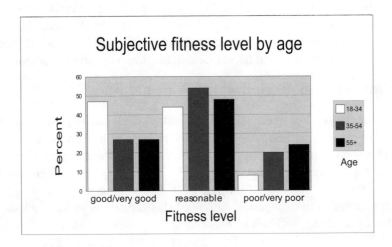

Figure 4.5: Gender differences in percieved fitness level

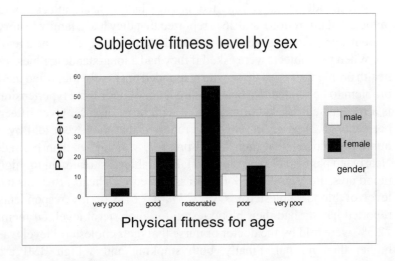

Healthy behaviours

Participants were asked to report whether they did anything to keep themselves healthy. Fifty-one per cent reported that they did do something and 49% that they did nothing. They were then asked to list

79

the three most important things they did to keep healthy. The three most popular health-promoting activities were taking exercise, eating healthy food and staying happy by occupying oneself mentally and physically. Other responses included reduction in smoking and alcohol, taking vitamin pills and taking treatments prescribed by the doctor.

Unhealthy behaviours

Participants were then asked to report if they did anything which involved risking their health and to list risky or unhealthy behaviours. Thirty-three per cent reported that they did risk their health whereas 66.7% reported that they did not. By far the most risky behaviour reported was smoking, followed by long working hours or dangers associated with occupation, and poor diet. Other responses included heavy drinking, and lack of exercise.

Heart disease, diabetes and chronic illness or disability

Four respondents (3%) reported having had a heart attack (or a myocardial infarction), and 26% reported that they had a family history (parents, brothers or sisters) of myocardial infarction under the age of 65. When the subjects were asked if they had a long-standing illness or health problem, 30% of those who responded positively identified their problem to be related to a heart or circulatory condition. Hypertension is a recognised risk factor associated with heart disease. Over fifteen per cent (15.2) of my respondents reported that they were told by a nurse or a doctor that their blood pressure was higher than normal. Nearly ten per cent (9.6%) reported taking tablets as treatment for high blood pressure. Another risk factor associated with heart disease is the level of blood cholesterol. Over 27% (27.6%) of my respondents reported having had their blood tested for cholesterol level. Of them, 22.5% were told by the doctor or nurse that their cholesterol level was higher than normal. Finally, both smoking and a high BMI are associated with heart disease. The BMI results were reported above. My study found that 25.5% of the respondents smoked daily, 6.7% were occasional smokers and 14.8% ex-smokers. The mean age for starting smoking was 18.2 years. The mean number of cigarettes smoked per day was 14.5.

Table 4.3: Heart disease: risk factors

Risk factor	%
Hypertension	15.2%
Blood cholesterol	22.5%
Smoking	32%

Four respondents (3%) reported that they were diabetics.(Nabarro (1988) reported that the age-adjusted prevalence of clinically diagnosed diabetes (all types) in England ranges between 1.05% and 1.36%.) When asked if they had a long-term illness, health problem or handicap 28.7% answered positively. The following list gives the nature of health problem as reported by 40 of the respondents.

Table 4.4: Reported long-term illness

	%
Heart or circulatory	30.0
Musculoskeletal	17.5
Respiratory	10.0
Skin problem	5.0
Sensory problem	5.0
Mental health problem	2.5
Other health problem	27.5
Cancer	2.5

Discussion of findings

Nearly half (48.8%) the women in the study and 35.9% of the men are overweight. This is a worrying statistic, especially when we consider that a third of the respondents are smokers, almost a quarter of those who were tested have been found to have raised cholesterol levels, and over 15% have hypertension. Although the incidence of myocardial infarction is similar to that reported by studies of the general population, the reported incidence of morbidity due to heart or circulatory disease is almost three times higher than that of the rest of the country. It is interesting to note that the Cyprus Department of Health reported that in 1993 the main cause of death amongst Greek Cypriots was due to cardiovascular diseases such as ischaemic heart disease and strokes. Although there are limitations in the findings of my study, they are, I believe, useful indicators of the health status of the Greek and Greek Cypriot community which need to be considered by those working in the health field.

As regards the other reported long-term illnesses, these seemed to correlate with the findings of a study of 93 Greek and Greek Cypriot women, which found that the most frequent cause of ill health was cardiovascular disease, followed by diseases of the musculoskeletal system such as arthritis and backache, followed by health problems associated with stress such as depression, tiredness, migraine and insomnia, followed by diseases of the respiratory system especially asthma (Papadopoulos and Worrall, 1996). The women in that study were asked to state whether in their opinion their health problems were associated with their occupation, past or present. Over a third reported positively, stating that sitting at the sewing machine for hours (commonly known as machining) meant that they took very little exercise and that this was the main reason for their becoming overweight. In their view, backache and pains in the shoulders and hands were also the result of machining. The relative isolation of the women who machine at home often results in depression. Some of the women in that study reported that their asthma was the cumulative effect of breathing the dust and chemicals from the clothes they machine. With the increase in asthma in the population of the UK, commonly thought due to atmospheric pollution, many Greek Cypriots who work in the traditional clothing industry, (often called 'sweat shops' because of the poor environmental and employment conditions) may be at further risk of developing asthma. While further studies will need to be undertaken to test this hypothesis, health and local authorities should undertake a campaign to promote health in the workplace.

The findings of this study reveal a variation in the way men and women define their health and fitness status. There is a marked tendency for the women to perceive these as reasonable (a mid-point in the scale used), whereas men's scores are more evenly spread. This may indicate either that women appear to be less satisfied with their health and fitness status than men or that they use a different conceptual framework to define health and fitness. Statistical testing revealed that there is a weak association between the way men, and women define their health status, and that the gender difference in fitness definition is statistically significant.

Section 3: Dietary habits

Respondents were asked to indicate the types of food they ate and how often they consumed them., as shown in *Table 4.5*. The majority of respondents (96%) reported that they ate red meat; more than a third of them (34.5%) eat it most days. The frequency of poultry consumption is high (45.5%), while the consumption of fish is low, particularly that of oily fish, with 27% of the respondents reporting that they rarely or never eat it. Over 15% reported eating fried foods most days. The frequent consumption of cakes, biscuits and hard as opposed to soft cheeses is a cause for concern. On the positive side, there is a high consumption of raw vegetables and fruit; on average, 75% of the sample reported eating these most days.

Table 4.5: Frequency of consumption of key food groups

	Most days	Once a week	Once/twice a month	Rarely or never
	%	%	%	%
Red Meat	34.5	51.7	9.7	4.1
Poultry	45.5	51.0	2.1	1.4
Processed meat	5.8	18.0	28.8	47.5
White fish	7.5	44.9	30.6	16.3
Oily fish	4.3	30.0	38.6	27.1
Rice, pasta, purguri	24.6	63.0	10.1	2.2
Raw vegetables	73.6	22.3	1.4	2.7
Boiled vegetables	44.8	43.4	5.6	6.3
Pulses	13.5	58.9	17.7	9.9
Fried foods	15.5	41.9	28.4	14.2
Fruit	77.0	18.2	2.0	2.7
Cakes,biscuits, sweets	43.0	39.4	9.9	7.7
Hard cheese (high fat)	43.6	37.6	13.4	5.4
Soft Cheese (low fat)	8.9	22.2	12.6	56.3
Low fat yogurt	20.3	33.1	15.8	30.8
Full fat yogurt	4.3	27.1	31.4	37.1

Respondents were particularly asked to report the frequency of consumption of bread, butter/margarine, milk and eggs.

Table 4.6: Foods eaten most frequently

	%
White bread/crackers/pitta	65.5
Wholemeal bread/crackers/pitta	32.4
Don't eat bread	2.1
Butter/Hard margarine	7.6
Polyunsaturated margarine	3.4
Low fat spread	64.8
Don't eat butter or margarine	17.9
	6.2
Whole/full cream milk	28.0
Semi-skimmed	60.6
Skimmed	9.1
Don't drink milk	2.3
Eggs per week	0-15 eggs (average 2.5)

The participants were asked if they ate traditional Greek foods like keftedes (fried meatballs), sheftalia (a type of sausage made with minced meat and wrapped in animal intestinal membrane which is normally quite fatty), kebabs and moussaka – all foods rich in animal fat–, and traditional vegetarian dishes such as fasolia (beans), louvi (black eye peas), and soups, and, if they did, how often. Over eighty seven per cent of the respondents (87.7%) reported that they ate the traditional meat dishes often or very often and 89.8% reported that they ate the traditional vegetarian dishes often or very often.

In order to summarise the different elements of the diet and relate these to recommended dietary intake, the food data were recoded to derive a dietary behaviour score. The method of scoring is based on the broadly accepted recommendation that a healthy diet should be low in fat, sugar and salt, and high in fibre (DHSS, 1984; HEA, 1991). More women are 'healthy eaters' than men. There was a weak to moderate positive correlation between healthy eating and those over 55 years in age. More first generation than second generation immigrants respondents were 'healthy eaters'; this was expected bearing in mind that all the over 55s belonged to this group. It seems that healthy eating may be related to the traditional Greek diet, but unfortunately I was unable to test this hypothesis not having any second generation over 55 year olds in my sample. Healthy eating was not related to income nor to education. However, the best knowledge about food was possessed by those in the 35–54 year old age group from both the first and second generation, while the over 55s appeared to know least. Finally, it is interesting to note that more women than men gained higher food knowledge scores, although this was not statistically significant.

Changes in diet

Respondents were asked whether they had changed their dietary habits during the previous year and, if they had, why. Just over twenty three per cent (23.3%) responded positively. The main reason for the change was to improve their health (35.7%), followed by the desire to improve their appearance (32.1%), for medical reasons (21.4%), and a variety of other reasons (10.7%). When asked if they thought they were eating a healthy diet, 68.8% reported that they did.

Discussion of findings

It is generally reported that the 'Mediterranean' diet, is a healthy diet. The traditional Greek diet is basically vegetarian with high consumption of raw vegetables and fruits, potatoes, pulses and cereals. It needs to be remembered that the populations of Greece and Cyprus were, until the 1960s, agricultural and that the soil and the weather of both these countries favours such crops. Animal farming was less common: sheep, goats and cows were kept to provide milk for daily consumption and for cheese making. Meat was expensive to buy and most families would eat it usually once or twice a week, mainly on Sundays. With the arrival of tourism and other industries in the last 30 years, more people have found full and better paid employment and therefore have been able to raise their standard of living; an important indicator of 'doing well' was both the increase in meat in the diet and a general increase in the volume of all foods. These changes have resulted in heart disease of epidemic proportions. This is confirmed by the 1991 Cyprus *Health and Hospital Statistics* and the 1995 report from the Cypriot department of Medical Services and Public Health. In August 1995, an article in the *Parikiaki*, the Greek newspaper of the community in the UK, reported that, according to the president of the Cypriot cardiac society, 2000 Greek Cypriots die every year from heart disease, while 600 Greek Cypriots are sent abroad to have cardiac surgery, costing the government millions of pounds; and all these for a country with a population of around 600,000 (Tokas, 1995). A common saying in Cyprus that reflects the realisation of the people that this is a negative and dangerous change is, 'We work as though we'll live forever and we eat as though we'll die tomorrow.' Most of the respondents in my study would hold similar values about food to those held by their compatriots living in Greece or Cyprus. The findings of my study indicate that, although more than two thirds of the respondents think that they eat a healthy diet (perhaps because they eat plenty of vegetables and fruit) their consumption of red meat, cakes and hard cheeses is too high. This finding helps to explain the previous finding that almost 50% of women and 36% of men are either slightly overweight or obese. These findings may also indicate that it not helpful to talk in blanket terms about how good or bad particular diets are. The meaning of a 'Mediterranean diet' for a food scientist, a TV cook, a nurse, a Greek, an Italian, and so on, may differ enormously, yet the generalisation that is often made in the popular press is that the 'Mediterranean diet' is healthy. The danger is that both health professionals, and people such as the Greeks pay less attention to this very important area of health behaviour.

It is worth noting that one of the Department of Health's (1992) targets included in the *Health of the Nation* strategy is that, by the year 2005, the proportion of obese men should be 6% and that of obese women only 8% of the population.

Section 4: Alcohol consumption

Twenty–six respondents (17.4%) reported that they never drank alcohol and 8.7% that they used to but no longer drink alcohol. The vast majority (59%) of my informants drink alcohol once a week and less than twice a month. A total of 14.8% consume alcohol between twice a week and every day. Ninety–eight respondents (89.1%) rated themselves as light drinkers and 10.9% rated themselves as moderate drinkers. Nobody rated him/herself a heavy drinker. When asked to report how many units of alcohol they consumed in a typical week including the weekend (using the 1992 HEA standard drink table), 95% of those who responded reported drinking between 0-10 units of alcohol. Only five respondents (5%) said they were drinking between 12–32 units. When asked if they thought their current level of alcohol consumption was harmful to their health, three respondents answered affirmatively (2.7%) and 107 (97.3%) answered negatively. Similarly, 95.5% did not wish to change their present level of alcohol consumption.

Respondents were asked to state what they thought were the safe alcohol limits for men and women. The ranges given for men were 0–100 units, the mean being 9.9 units of alcohol. The ranges given for women were 0–50 units, the mean being 7.6 units of alcohol.

Figure 4.6: Alcohol consumption by age per week

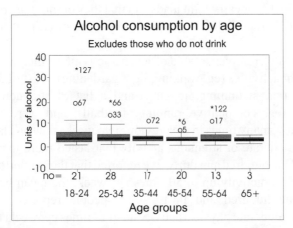

Discussion on findings

The findings of my study are in stark contrast to the findings of Theodorou (1992); in her study of 160 interviews of Cypriots (Greek and Turkish) carried out in North London, she found that the level of harmful consumption (over 35 units per week) in the Cypriot community is considerably higher than that of the overall population. She found that 48.8% of the men and 12.6% of the women in the sample drank more than 35 units per week. This may be explained by the fact that she used a 'snowball' sample, whereas mine was a random sample. Theodorou used semi-structured interviews to obtain her data, whereas I used a postal questionnaire. Methodological problems and biases associated with these methods of data collection are well documented. Another study is needed to confirm or refute either of these findings in order to enable health providers and purchasers to make appropriate decisions.

Section 5: Activity at work and leisure

Respondents were asked to describe the type and level of physical activity they undertook on a daily basis either at work or at home. A large proportion, 42.9%, reported that they are usually sitting and do not walk about much, while a slightly smaller percentage, 38.6%, reported that they stand or walk quite a lot but their work or housework does not involve heavy lifting. An even smaller number, 15% , reported that they usually lift or carry light loads and that they climb stairs often, and finally 3.6% reported that they do heavy work or carry heavy loads often.

Subjects were given a table of leisure activities which contained a list of light activities (eg. walking, light gardening), a list of moderate activities (eg. swimming, jogging) and a list of strenuous leisure activities (eg. competitive running, football), and were asked to indicate how many times in the previous two weeks they had taken part in light, moderate or strenuous activity that lasted more than twenty minutes. One hundred and thirty five reported that they undertook some light physical activity up to 50 times per week, the mean being 6.37 times. One hundred and thirty seven people reported that they undertook moderate physical activity up to 12 times per week, the mean being 1.61 times. One hundred and seven reported that they had not undertaken any strenuous leisure activity in the previous two weeks. Twenty–two reported undertaking such activity between one and five times, six reported undertaking strenuous leisure activity between six and ten times and two reported it to be more than ten times.

In order to assess the levels of activity of my sample, activity scales were constructed. These scales replicate those of the Allied Dunbar National Fitness Survey (ADNFS) (Sports Council,1992). The ADNFS recommended that individuals should participate in at least three sessions of a mix of moderate and vigorous activity per week, each lasting a minimum of twenty minutes in order to confer cardiovascular benefits. The scales used in this survey replicated those of the ADNFS but have been adjusted to a two week period (*Table 4.7*).

Table 4.7: Activity level scales based on activity in previous two weeks

Level 5:	Six or more occasions of vigorous activity
Level 4:	Six or more occasions mixed between moderate and vigorous activity
Level 3:	Six or more occasions of moderate activity
Level 2:	Three to five occasions of mixed moderate or vigorous activity
Level 1:	One to two occasions of mixed moderate or vigorous activity
Level 0:	No occasions of moderate or vigorous activity

Of the 139 cases for whom data was available only 10% achieved their target activity level as defined by ADNFS. There was no correlation between the sexes as to whether they reached their target level. However, reaching one's target level was correlated with age. More of the 18–34 year olds reached their target level (n=9 out of 58) compared with those in the 35–54 age group (n=3 out of 53) and those in the 55+ age group (n=2 out of 28). Of those who reached their target level, 71% said their fitness was good or very good compared with only 32% of those who did not reach their target level. None of those who described their health as reasonable, poor or very poor, reached their target level compare with 12% of those who described their health as good or very good.

Asked whether they felt they took enough exercise for someone of their age, 48 responded yes, and 102 responded no. Those who responded negatively were asked to state what prevents them taking more exercise. The results are presented in *Table 4.8.*

Table 4.8: Reasons preventing respondents taking more exercise

	%
Lack of time	56.8
Lack of motivation	38.7
Lack of money	25.2
Illness or disability	15.3
Lack of transport	10.8
Lack of accessible facilities at work	9.9
Lack of accessible facilities in the community	9.9
Other reasons	8.1

*Respondents could tick more than one box, therefore number > 100

Participants were asked to compare their current levels of activity with the levels of the previous year. Of those who responded, 18.6% stated that they were now more active, 60% stated that their activity levels were the same and 20.7% reported no change.

The two top reasons cited in *Table 4.8* were analysed further. I discovered that more of those who were fully occupied (in full employment, self employed, on a government employment scheme, or looking after home and children under the age of 16) gave 'lack of time' as their reason for not taking more exercise, compared with those who were not fully occupied (working fewer than 30 hours per week, waiting to start a job, unemployed or full time students). More men than women said they 'lacked motivation' (53% versus 33%). More of those who were fully occupied (definition as above) also reported lack of motivation compared with those not fully occupied (51% versus 29%); it was also found that the over 55 year olds were more likely to cite lack of motivation as a reason for not taking more exercise. However, there was no association between marital status and lack of motivation and this was irrespective of generation.

Asked if they would like to do more exercise and what type of activities they would most like to take part in, 47 reported that they would like to undertake a variety of activities such as aerobics, weight lifting, other gym activities etc, 43 stated that they would like to take part in or do more swimming, 32 would like to partake in more outdoor sports such as walking and cycling, 16 wish to be involved with football, tennis and badminton.

In order to account for levels of activity that respondents engaged in at work or during usual (non-leisure) daytime activities, a new variable was constructed which combined this activity and the leisure time activities. Those who reported that they usually sit and do not walk much were assigned a score of 0 (see activity level scales, *Table 4.7*). Those who reported that they stand or walk about quite a lot but do not carry or lift things were assigned a score of 2. Those whose work involved climbing often and/or lifting light loads were assigned a score of 3. Those whose work involved heavy work or carrying heavy loads were assigned a score of 4. The activity scale was divided into three categories: 'sedentary' (a maximum of one or two occasions of moderate or vigorous activity; levels 0 and 1), 'active' (three to five occasions of mixed moderate and vigorous activity or six occasions of moderate but not vigorous activity; levels 2 and 3) and 'very active' (levels 4 and 5; six or more occasions of mixed moderate and vigorous activity). *Table 4.9* gives the results of this combined activity level for all the one hundred and twenty nine people for whom data were available. It points out that 60.5% of the respondents were found to be sedentary which is a worrying statistic.

Table 4.9: Combined activity level scores (n=129)

Category	N	%
Sedentary	78	60.5
Active	34	26.4
Very Active	17	13.2

The most sedentary were found to be the over 55 year olds, more likely to be women than men or those with a chronic illness or disability and the overweight.

Participants were asked to express their opinions on ten statements about exercise. The results from those who responded are reported in *Table 4.10*.

Table 4.10: Respondents' views about exercise (n=147)

	Agree %	Not sure %	Disagree %
Vigorous exercise can be dangerous if you are not used to it	78.9	19.0	2.1
Sport is only for fit, young people	12.7	15.5	71.8
Regular exercise is important if you want to lose weight	80.4	16.1	3.5
Exercising outdoors is better for you than exercising indoors	31.0	34.5	34.5
Regular exercise can help reduce your risk of heart disease	81.5	15.8	2.7
You need a lot of expensive equipment to get fit	4.3	28.0	58.0
Regular exercise makes you look more masculine	14.0	28.0	58.0
A short walk a day is better than no exercise at all	90.5	6.8	2.7
Pregant women should not exercise	7.6	31.0	61.4
You can't get fit on your own	9.2	18.3	72.5

In order to measure the participants' knowledge about exercise all the above views (with the exception of 'regular exercise makes you look more masculine') were given a score of 3 for the correct response, a score of 2 for 'not sure/it depends' and a score of 1 for the incorrect response. Although overall, Greek Cypriots appear to have a fairly good knowledge about exercise, the results showed that individuals from the first generation and those who were aged 55 and over had the lowest knowledge. There was no difference between the sexes. Those scoring high tended to be those with college and university education. However, a good knowledge about exercise did not result in higher levels of activity and there was no association between good knowledge and the achievement of the target level of exercise. Good knowledge did not result in better motivation for more activity.

Discussion of findings

The Royal College of Physicians (1991), reported that regular exercise helps reduce the risk of heart disease, helps control mild hypertension and protects against the onset of osteoporosis in women. Steinberg and Sykes (1993) also found that exercise is beneficial to mental health. Probably the most significant findings from my study are that 60% of the sample lead sedentary lives and that only 10% of them achieved their target activity level. The women, the overweight, the over 55 year olds, the first generation Greek Cypriots, and those who suffer from a chronic illness appear to be the most at risk. The findings pointed towards an association between lower levels of activity and knowledge, and individuals who were classified as first generation; all the indicators pointed towards a link between culture and exercise, but I was unable to test this hypothesis as there were no respondents who were over 55 in the second generation category. My findings are worse than the national average as reported by the *Health Survey for England 1994* (Colhoun and Prescott-Clark, 1996) which found that just under 18% of their sample were classified as inactive or sedentary. Clearly this is an area that merits further investigation among the Greek Cypriot community; closer involvement of the community would also result in more effective health promotion initiatives.

Section 6: Smoking

As mentioned earlier, a total of 32% of my respondents are smokers. Of them, 25% stated that they smoke daily, and 7% occasionally. Fifteen per cent reported that they were ex-smokers, but a 53% majority had never smoked. The age for starting smoking ranged between 9 years and 38 years. Those who smoke daily smoke between 2 and 30 cigarettes, or up to 17 cigars, or up to 0.2 ounces of tobacco. Informants were asked whether they would like to alter their smoking behaviour: 32.6% reported that they were happy to stay smoking the same amount, 21.7% would like to cut down a bit, 8.7% would like to cut down a lot, and 37% wished to give it up altogether. The findings did not reveal any correlations between smoking and age, levels of stress, levels of alcohol consumption, education or level of exercise.

Respondents were asked whether they thought the amount they smoked was harmful to their health. Over seventy-eight per cent (78.3%) responded positively and 21.7% negatively. They were also asked whether they had, in the previous 12 months, made a serious attempt to give up smoking. Over a quarter (26.7%) answered positively and 73.3% negatively. Those who had tried to stop reported that they had started again because they lacked the will power (30%), because they were stressed or bored (20%) and for other reasons (50%). However, 47.7% reported that they had cut down the amount they smoked during the previous 12 months.

Table 4.11: Ex-smokers' reasons for giving up smoking

	Very Important %	Fairly Important %	Not Important %
Felt it was bad for own health	13.9	83.4 *	—
Costing too much money	26.3	36.8	36.8
Advice from a doctor or nurse	58.8	11.8	29.4
Pressure from family or friends	35.3	17.6	47.1
Felt it was antisocial	14.3	42.9	42.9
Not allowed to smoke at work	—	7.1	92.9

In answer to the question 'Do any of the members of your household smoke?', 50.3% of those who responded reported positively, and 49.7% responded negatively. Of those who answered positively, 56 reported that there was one member of the household who smoked, ten reported that two members smoked, four that three members smoked and two reported that four members of their household smoked.

Respondents were asked to indicate how many cigarettes a day a person would have to smoke before risking their health. The answer of the majority of the respondents was between 1 and 5 cigarettes; 31 answered between 6 and 10 cigarettes and almost as many thought that one had to smoke between 11 and 20 cigarettes before risking health; a further 15 thought that one would need to smoke 21–30 cigarettes per day before risking one's health and the remaining eight reported this to be 31 and over cigarettes per day.

Participants were asked to express their views on a number of statements related to smoking restrictions.

Table 4.12: Respondents views about smoking restrictions

	More restrictions %	About the same %	Fewer restrictions %
On buses	58.5	35.4	5.4
On trains	60.5	36.1	4.1
On aeroplanes	67.1	26.6	6.3
In restaurants and cafes	59.6	33.6	6.8
In cinemas and theatres	59.7	32.6	7.6
In banks and post offices	63.2	33.3	3.5
In all shops	63.4	31.7	4.8
In public houses	52.8	37.5	9.7
In hospitals and clinics	74.7	20.5	4.8
In all enclosed public places	71.0	23.4	5.5
In all public places	49.7	39.2	11.2
In places where you work or study	60.0	32.4	7.6

Participants were asked to say whether or not the smoke from cigarettes could be harmful to the health of non- smokers who breathe it regularly. Of those who responded, one hundred and thirty one reported that passive smoking was harmful to adults, while one hundred and forty four said that this was harmful to children and babies.

Discussion of findings

The Health Education Authority (HEA, 1994) reported that the highest smoking prevalence amongst minority ethnic groups (Afro-Caribbean, Indian, Pakistani and Bangladeshi) was that of the Banlgadeshis at 23%. As already discussed in section 2, smoking is one of the major risk factors for heart disease. The findings of my study show that compared with the whole population in England smoking in the Greek Cypriot community is higher by 2%, and by 9% compared with other minority ethnic groups. Judging by their various responses the Greek Cypriot smokers realise that both active and passive smoking is bad for their health. However, only just over a quarter of them attempted to give it up, the majority of whom were unsuccessful. Advice from a health professional seems to be the most significant deterrent.

The Department of Health has set a number of targets in its *Health of the Nation* strategy which need to be achieved by the year 2000. One of these is to reduce the prevalence of cigarette smoking to no more than

20% by the year 2000 in both men and women. The findings of this survey suggest that unless urgent and co-ordinated action is taken using the 'healthy alliance model' (involvement of statutory health and social services sectors as well as the voluntary sector), it is highly unlikely that the DoH targets on smoking will be achieved within the Greek Cypriot community.

Section 7: Stress

Respondents were asked to indicate how stressful their lives were at the time of completing the questionnaire. A 10 point scale was used with the score of 1 being 'not at all stressful' and 10 as 'very stressful'. Twenty–one per cent of the sample reported that their lives were relatively stressless by scoring 1–4; some 16% rated their stress at level 5, the mid–point of the scale that indicated that they are fairly stressed.The overwhelming majority (64%) reported themselves to be under a lot of stress by rating their stress between 6 and 10.

The ten point stress level scale was dichotomised at level 6: level 1–5 was assigned as 'low' stress and 6+ as 'high'. This new variable was used to explore differences in stress levels between age groups and between men and women. There was no relationship found between stress level and gender but there were differences between age groups: lower proportions of those aged 55+ were found to have high stress levels (41% versus 70% of those aged 35–54, and 68% of those age 18–34). Level of stress was also cross–tabulated with a number of other variables: reported income, social activity, health perceptions, marital status, whether they had children or not, whether fully occupied or not, and generation of the respondents. These were not found to be associated or, if they were, the findings were not statistically significant. However, there was an association between stress level and level of happiness: 83% of those who were unhappy had high stress levels (6+) compared with 52% of those who described themselves as 'happy/very happy').

Participants were asked to list their three greatest causes of stress in descending order of magnitude. Work was most frequently cited as the respondents' greatest cause of stress (40%) followed by family (12%) and financial problems (12%). Ten per cent cited their own health or the health of others as their greatest cause of stress. Unemployment and loneliness were cited by 5% of the respondents. The second greatest causes of stress that respondents reported were family issues or problems (25%), financial concerns (20%), work (11%), own health or health of others (8%), and unemployment, loneliness and isolation (5%). A number of other specific reasons, too many to form categories, were given.

The data on stressors were explored for differences between men and women and age groups. There was no association found between gender and stressors but a moderate association was found between age and type of stressor. As *Figure 4.7* illustrates, those aged under 55 gave work as their greatest cause of stress, whereas those aged 55+ most frequently gave their own health or the health of others as their greatest cause of stress. Family concerns were equally spread throughout the age groups whereas financial concerns were greater among those aged 35–54. Loneliness or isolation was cited as the greatest cause of stress only by those who were aged 55+.

Figure 4.7: Greatest causes of stress by age groups

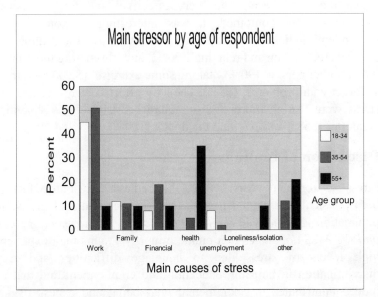

Participants were asked their views about a number of behaviours which are commonly cited as 'stress reducers' or responses to high levels of stress.

Table 4.13: Opinions of respondents on a number of behaviours and their effectiveness in reducing stress

	Very effective %	Fairly effective %	Not at all effective %
Trying to forget your problems	24.1	40.9	35.0
Resting and relaxing	55.9	40.0	4.1
Having a few drinks	10.2	36.5	53.3
Having a cigarette	11.0	23.5	65.4
Visiting the doctor	4.3	35.5	60.1
Taking some exercise	34.0	48.2	17.7
Eating more	7.4	14.7	77.9
Taking tablets	7.3	20.4	72.3
Spending money	13.9	29.9	56.2
Discussing the problem with another person	52.1	37.5	10.4

When the results from the 'very effective' and fairly effective' categories were combined, it was interesting to note that the respondents believed that the most effective ways for dealing with stress were: 'resting and relaxing' (96%), and 'discussing the problem with another person' (90%), 'taking some exercise' (82%) and 'trying to forget your problems' (65%). The least effective ways for reducing stress were 'eating more' (78%), 'taking tablets' (72%), 'having a cigarette' (65%) and 'visiting the doctor' (60%).

Discussion of findings

Stress has, for many years, been established as a contributory factor to both physical and mental illness. In 1995 the Health of the Nation publication *Variations in Health. What can the Department of Health and the NHS do?* states that ethnic minority groups may experience high levels of stress due to language difficulties and racial discrimination in housing, education and employment and that this indeed contributes to poor mental well–being and excess risks of coronary heart disease.

The respondents in this study have reported high levels of stress due mainly to work, family and financial reasons. The higher stress levels reported by those in the age group of 18–34 years and 35–54 may be due to these groups having the whole range of 'work profile'. Those at the lower end of the age scale would probably be trying to enter the job market and may be finding this difficult, or if they have gained employment are trying to adjust to new life patterns and relationships. Those in the middle of the age scale may have found themselves in dead end, poorly paid jobs and may be facing economic difficulties, having to support a family. Those at the top end of the age scale may be facing redundancy, or more likely for a Greek Cypriot man, bankruptcy. All these work scenarios would also explain the financial difficulties and even the family problems.

Another explanation for the high stress levels being attributed to family reasons may be that of the generation gap. Unlike the accepted or even expected practice within the indigenous population, whereby children often leave the family home when they reach adulthood, Greek parents expect to care for their children who will stay with them until they are married. It is likely that the 'parents' in this study would be first generation Greek/Greek Cypriots, who hold different values from their children. Family problems may also be the result of changing roles between husband and wife. Greek women are expected to clean the house, do the laundry, cook the dinner, look after the children and even the friends and relatives who will call or visit from Cyprus, as well as going to work or working from home. And although men can go out on their own or with their friends, women are prohibited from similar pursuits not because they need their husbands' permission but simply because they were brought up to believe that 'good women' do not have the need to go out on their own. However, circumstances, if not changes in traditions, are sometimes forcing couples to realise that the expectations they have from each other do not match and this may result in conflict and raised levels of stress.

Fernando (1991) explains that coping with stress is related to cultural values and that coping practices cannot be considered in isolation from culture. In Western psychology, coping with stress is usually perceived in behavioural terms, consisting of cognitive processes, such as denial, repression and intellectualisation.This, however, ignores the cultural context in which coping occurs and the way coping is perceived and judged in a racist milieu. Therefore culture plays a large part in determining the way in which a particular event of emotional distress is conceptualised, for example, whether it is seen as 'illness' to be cured or endured (coping), or as a spiritual crisis to be resolved or experienced (understanding). Coping strategies have been categorised by Folkman and Lazarus (1988) as 'problem-focused' and 'emotion-focused': the former is geared to resolving the problem and the latter directed at reducing distress, irrespective of its underlying cause. Both forms of coping are necessary, but the effectiveness of coping in any given situation depends on the appropriateness of the choice between the two. Greeks and Greek Cypriots are regarded as 'Southern European' or 'Mediterranean' and are therefore usually excluded from discussions on ethnic health. The emphasis in research and in service provision has always been with 'New Commonwealth' immigrants and their families, which if strictly interpreted, of course, includes Cypriots, but which in practice has become a euphemism for the Black ethnic minorities whom British society has regarded as having the greatest difficulties in settling and living here (Littlewood, 1988). However, while Greeks and Greek Cypriots base many of their conceptual and ideological frameworks on 'Western' foundations (it could be said that some of these foundations have their roots in the ancient Greek civilisation, such as medicine), those living in Britain share with Black groups many difficulties and characteristics such as language problems, their own unique cultural ideologies and practices, experience of racism/discrimination, problems of identity particularly amongst the second and subsequent generations, and so on.

Constantinides (1988) identified an urgent need for information on the epidemiology of mental health and stress-related illness in the Greek communities; this need still exists in 1996, and service planning continues to take place largely in a vacuum. Furthermore, GPs and hospital staff need training in the issues affecting the Greek communities, but not in a manner which would create stereotypes, which in turn could breed prejudice or encourage a simplistic perception of problems.

Section 8: Home, family and social life

Social support systems

Respondents were asked to say whether they had anyone they could count on when they needed to talk over problems or make difficult decisions. Eighty–six per cent reported they did indeed have someone. More women reported having a confidant (93% versus 75%).

There was no association between having a confidant and age, marital status or whether first or second generation.

Respondents who reported that they had a confidant were asked to state who it was that they confided in. Just over 41% reported that they confided in their spouses or partners. Almost one third (30.8%) reported that they could discuss their problems with more than one person; just over fourteen per cent (14.4%) reported that they talked to a female family member; one tenth (9.6%) stated that they depended on friends or colleagues; some three per cent (2.9%) shared their problems with a male member of the family and 1% gave various other answers. Single people (including divorcees and the widowed) were more likely to talk to family members or colleagues. They were also more likely to confide in more than one person. Older or married/cohabiting respondents were more likely to confide in their spouse/ partner.

Caring responsibilities

Participants were asked to indicate whether they or other members of the household were caring for anyone suffering from long–standing physical illness, mental handicap or mental illness. They were further asked to state the age of the person for whom they were caring. This was reported to be between 8 years old and 88 years old.

Table 4.14: Respondents' caring responsibilities

	Yes %	No %
Long standing physical illness	8.8	91.2
Mental handicap	0.8	99.2
Mental illness	4.6	95.4

Social activities

Participants were asked to indicate how often they have visitors or go out to, for example, social clubs, eating out, religious meetings, or visiting friends and family. The vast majority, (71.8%) reported that they socialised about once a week. Almost twenty three per cent (22.5%) reported that they socialised at least once a month, and 5.6% reported that they took part in such social activities less than once a month or never.

Almost eighty per cent (79.6%) of the participants reported that they either never or very infrequently did any voluntary work. Nearly twelve per cent (11.7%) reported that they had been involved in some form of voluntary work at least once a month, 6.6% stated that they did voluntary work once a week, only 2.2% reported to have been involved daily. Nearly 7% reported having been involved in fund raising while the others (93%) reported a number of various activities.

Respondents were asked to state whether they were generally satisfied with their social lives. Some 14.4% reported to be very satisfied, 65.1% to be satisfied and 20.5% reported to be dissatisfied. More men than women reported being very satisfied (23% versus 9%). Dissatisfaction with social life was more common among those aged 35–54 (33% versus 12% of 18–34 year olds and 16% of those aged 55+, p=.052). Those who were single, widowed and divorced more frequently stated they were dissatisfied with their social life (27% versus 16%). Dissatisfaction was also more common among first generation respondents (28% versus 12%), and among those on a low income (30% versus 13%).

Respondents were also asked to say how happy they usually felt. The vast majority (65.5%) reported being happy, 6.2% stated they were very happy, while 28.2% reported they were 'not very happy' or 'very unhappy'. The data were further explored to look at the associations with stress levels, health/chronic illness, and levels of happiness. More of those with high stress levels (6+) were dissatisfied with their social life (27% versus 12%) as were those who were in poor health or chronically ill (34% versus 16%). More than half (58%) of those who were 'not very happy/very unhappy' felt dissatisfied compared with 8% of those who were 'happy/very happy'.

Discussion of findings

The findings of this study indicate that Greek Cypriots enjoy fairly good social support systems and family networks. The existence of such networks are of immense importance and are closely associated with levels of stress and health. As this study has shown, those who were isolated were more likely to be dissatisfied with their social life and were more likely to be unhappy and to suffer higher stress levels. Naturally, this is a complex phenomenon for which it would be difficult to isolate a cause and effect relationship. Helman (1990) reports that several authors have noted the importance of social support, at all stages of life, in protecting against stress which can give rise to physical and behavioural abnormalities (Weinman, 1981; Brown and Harris, 1979; Kiritz and Moos, 1974). The Greek Cypriot community in North London remains a close knit community. Even though the cultural and social cohesion is constantly adapting and changing, it appears that even second and third generation Greek Cypriots retain their 'Greekness' or Cypriotness'. Furthermore, it is my belief, based on my membership of and work with the community, that the second generation men and women continue to be very interested in our culture and are slowly becoming involved in activities that promote the interests of our community.

The levels of volunteering is somewhat disappointing but, as I pointed out in the previous paragraph, this is gradually changing. However, it is worth pointing out that a definition of 'voluntary work' was not given in the questionnaire and this may have led to inconsistent responses. The respondents may have perceived volunteering as something formal such as working for the Samaritans, Cancer Research, or other well known voluntary organisations. At a more informal level, taking a neighbour to the hospital, shopping for a house boundfriend or neighbour, helping at one's child's/children's school, may not be perceived as voluntary work but as an act of kindness or just being helpful. Traditionally, many first generation Greek Cypriots involved themselves (and still do) in associations that individuals from different Cypriot villages formed in order to maintain social networks, friendships and their villages' memories and traditions. These self-help associations exist purely through voluntary membership and their maintenance requires a lot of voluntary activities; this type of activity may not be viewed as volunteering but as socialising activities. This lack of clarity may have influenced the findings. Volunteering, it seems, is not part of our culture. This is an area that is gradually being addressed.

Section 9: Respondents' health and their use of health services

GP consultations

Respondents were asked to report the last time they consulted their family doctor (GP).

Table 4.15: When was the last time you saw your GP?

	%	(N)
Less than 1 week ago	14.8	(22)
Less than 1 month ago	26.8	(40)
Less than 3 months ago	24.8	(37)
Less than 6 months ago	14.1	(21)
Less than 1 year ago	14.1	(21)
Less than 5 years ago	3.4	(5)
Never	2.0	(3)

Respondents were asked about the method of their last consultation with their GP. One hundred and forty three people (96.6%) reported that they last saw their GP in his/her surgery. One person (0.7%) reported speaking to the GP over the telephone and four persons (2.7%) stated that they were visited at home.

Use of Accident and Emergency (A&E) departments

Participants were asked to report the number of times that they had visited the A&E department in the previous 12 months. Most of the respondents (79.7%) reported that they had not used the A&E department in the previous 12 months. Nineteen people (13.3%) had used it once, six (4.2%) had used it twice, two (1.4%) had used it three times, one (0.7%) had used it five times and one (0.7%) had used it nine times, as *Table 4.16* indicates.

Table 4.16: Reasons for attending the A&E department

Following an accident	34%
Referred by the GP	27%
Unable to see my GP	23%
Other	16%

Men were more likely to have attended an A&E department in the previous year than women (27% versus 16%). Other correlates of attending A&E were explored: those with high stress levels (6+) were more likely to have attended (26% versus 10%) irrespective of whether they were suffering from chronic illness/poor health. Those who were very satisfied with their social life, who also socialised more frequently, were more likely to have attended (40% versus 16% of those who were satisfied and 21% of those who were not satisfied).

Use of private medicine

Informants were asked whether they, or any member of their family, use private doctors and why. Of the 132 people who answered this question 46 (34.8%) replied positively. *Table 4.17* indicates the reasons for paying to see the doctor.

Table 4.17: Reasons for ucing private medicine *

I wanted a second opinion	n=22
I could not see my doctor when I needed to	n=11
My doctor does not believe I am ill	n=5
My doctor would not perscribe the test I thought I needed	n-4
My doctor does not understand me	n=4
My doctor would not perscribe the medicine I thought I needed	n=3
Other reasons	n=15

* (Numbers do not add up to 46 as some respondents gave more than one reason)

The data were explored to identify factors associated with the use of private medicine. Age, sex and generation were not associated. Those with high stress levels more frequently reported using private medicine and this was statistically significant (39% versus 27% [p-.17]). The only income group who did not use private medicine in significant numbers were those who had a personal income of £2.5K to £4K (the second lowest income group): only 17% of this group used private medicine compared with 33% or more of the other income groups.

Use of screening/ health 'check ups' within primary care

Individuals were asked whether they were likely to use health promotion services if they were available at their GP surgery or the health centre. Eighty-two per cent replied positively. They were then asked whether they were invited by their family doctor to attend for a routine health check in the previous 12 months. Over twelve per cent (12.8%) replied positively while a staggering 87.2% replied negatively. Over ninety per cent (90.5%) of those who replied positively reported that they had attended for their check up. Of those who attended, 47.4% reported that the check up was performed by their own doctor, 42.1% were seen by a nurse and 10.5% by another doctor. The one person who did not attend stated that s/he had no health problem and therefore no reason to attend.

Individuals were asked whether, during the preceding year, they had received advice from any of the members of the primary health team on a range of health issues, the results of which are reported in *Table 4.18* below.

Table 4.18: Areas of advice given by members of primary health care team

	Doctor %	Nurse %	Other %
Take more exercise	42.3	19.2	38.5
Cut down or give up alcohol	40.0	None	60.0
Cut down or give up smoking	59.1	None	40.9
Change diet	42.9	3.6	53.5
Lose weight	51.9	7.6	40.7
Rest or relax more often	63.2	5.3	31.5
Get a better night's sleep	42.3	3.8	53.8
Use condoms when having sex	16.7	33.3	50.0

Individuals were asked if they had ever had their blood pressure measured and if so when. Nearly ninety per cent (88.8%) reported that they had. Most of my subjects (53.7%) reported that their blood pressure was measured in the last six months, 17.9% reported it to have been between seven and twelve months, 24.4% between one and three years, 1.6 % between three and five years and 2.4% reported that their blood pressure was measured more than five years ago. Just over 15%

had been told by their doctor or the practice nurse that their blood pressure was higher than normal and 9.6% reported taking tablets for their hypertension.

Respondents were asked whether they had ever had their blood cholesterol level measured and if so when. Nearly thirty per cent (27.6%) reported that they had. Most of them (41%) reported that the test was done between seven and twelve months previously, equal numbers (23.1%) reported having had it done either six months or one to three years previously. Nearly thirteen per cent (12.8%) reported that they had had the test three to five years previously. Just over twenty-two per cent (22.5%) reported that they were told their blood cholesterol level was higher than normal.

Health screening for women

Seventy five per cent of the women participants reported that the surgery they were registered with had a woman GP on the team. All the women participants reported that they could see a female doctor on the same day for an emergency, for a booked appointment, for family planning advice, for a cervical smear test and for other women's health problems. Seventy six per cent of the women reported that they had been invited to have a cervical smear test, most of them reporting having had their test either during the previous six months (30.4%), or between one and three years previously (30.4%). Nearly sixteen per cent (15.9%) had their test during the previous seven and twelve months, 13% between three and five years and 10.1% over five years previously. In relation to breast cancer screening, only 23.6% of the women reported having had a mammogram or similar test. Some 5.6% were not sure whether they had been screened or not. Of those who responded positively equal numbers had had it done between one and three years previously (28.6%) and more than three but less than five years previously (28.6%). Nearly 10% had had it done more than five years previously, while the rest ranged between less than six months and between seven and twelve months.

Discussion of findings

This section of the survey included questions on the 'use of A&E departments' and 'use of private medicine'. The first area was designed to test the commonly held assumption by many professional health carers that Greek Cypriots abuse the Accident and Emergency departments either with minor complaints or instead of waiting to see their own GP. The survey revealed that only six respondents used the A& E because they were unable to see their GP and a further five gave their reason as 'other'. This is a very low figure and does not sustain the assumptions of those working or managing the Accident and Emergency departments; this is a clear illustration of stereotyping, the possible effects of which were discussed in a previous chapter.

The second area was testing evidence that I had obtained from the Greek Cypriots whom I interviewed and some that I did not, but had met socially; many had reported to me that for a variety of reasons they often paid to see a doctor. This assumption appears to be more sustainable. A fair number (46 out of 132 of those who responded), have used a 'private doctor'. The most frequent reason for this was that the respondents wanted to have a second opinion, which must mean a lack of trust in their GPs. Two other reasons ('my doctor does not believe I am ill' and 'my doctor does not understand me') indicate the lack of communication between doctor and patient. This finding has been consistently highlighted in the literature over the last two decades and it is further discussed in *Chapter 7*. Some of the reasons given for paying a 'private doctor' could be the reaction to racist behaviour by the staff. McNaught (1987) reported that ethnic minority patients were kept waiting unnecessarily, that they received poor or no explanation of treatment or care, that staff assumed that minority patients were 'faking' or were hypochondriacs, that treatments were delayed or inappropriate and that patients were denied medicine on the grounds that they had low pain thresholds. The recent survey on the health and lifestyles of black and minority ethnic groups in England by the Health Education Authority (1994) also supports these findings.

In respect of health 'check ups', it is encouraging to see that the uptake is high. However, there needs to be acknowledged that, particularly among the first generation Greek Cypriots, the attitude of ' I have no health problem and therefore no reason to go for tests' still exists. Bouri (1992) also reported this attitude in her study about breast cancer amongst the Greek Cypriot women. The community itself, through its various organisations is beginning to have some impact in this area but much work needs to be done.

Section 10: Views about health and causes of ill health

Heart disease

Participants were asked a series of questions about the causes of and beliefs regarding heart disease. Firstly they were asked to select one of the following statements which was closest with their point of view.

Table 4.19: Beliefs about heart attacks

	Agree %
Heart attacks can strike for no reason, they just happen. It's chance, fate, or plain bad luck	5.6
There are reasons why people have heart attacks but we can do nothing about them, for instance, they are inherited, or happen for reasons we don't understand	12.0
There are some steps you can take that might help to cut down your chance of a heart attack	42.4
You can definitely reduce your chances of having a heart attack if you follow the right advice	32.8
Heart attacks could be avoided completely if only we lived our lives in the right way	7.2

Eighteen per cent of respondents agreed with the first two statements which express a fatalistic view about the capacity to prevent heart attacks occurring. The majority (75%) had a more realistic view in believing that the individual has the potential for reducing their risk of heart attack, and 7% had an idealistic view.

Respondents were then presented with twenty factors and asked to rate their importance in relation to their contribution to the risk of having a heart attack. (*Table 4.20*)

Table 4.20: Respondents' opinions about risk factors for heart attacks

	Very important %	Important %	Not at all important %
High blood pressure	80.3	17.6	2.1
Fluoride in the water	2.6	19.7	77.8
Eating too much	82.2	15.8	2.1
Smoking cigarettes	75.5	19.6	4.9
Suffering from a sudden shock	39.1	53.6	7.2
Air pollution	18.3	42.0	39.7
Hard work	31.4	46.0	22.6
Not taking enough exercise	42.7	46.2	11.2
Stress/stenochoria	71.8	26.1	2.1
Being overweight	72.0	25.2	2.8
Family history	56.1	38.8	5.0
Being diabetic	15.9	40.2	43.9
Unemployed	7.4	35.6	57.0
Not getting enough sleep	5.9	31.1	63.0
Using too much salt	24.3	48.5	27.2
Loneliness	8.8	28.7	62.5
Drinking coffee	2.3	37.9	59.8
Drinking too much alcohol	33.1	51.1	15.8
Not having enough money	7.5	36.8	55.6
Taking the oral contraceptive pill	1.5	26.2	72.3

In order to identify which respondents were most knowledgeable about the contributory risk factors to heart disease a new variable was constructed: each of the responses to the 20 variables in the above table were assigned a score of 1 to 3. This score was then dichotomised at the median, a high score indicating more accurate knowledge. This variable was then cross–tabulated with a number of independent variables (gender, age, education and income). Overall there were no statistically significant associations. Although there was no pattern in the degree of knowledge between age groups, those aged 65+ were more likely to have a low level of knowledge with only 10% getting a high score compared with 54% of those aged 55–64. Those with a higher education more frequently had high knowledge scores (59% versus 50% of the those who attended college and 35% of those who had a secondary education).

Effects of behaviour on health

The participants in my study were asked to express their views about the possible effects of a number of behaviours on health. A series of questions was asked around diet, alcohol, smoking and stress. The results are presented in *Tables 4.21, 4.22, 4.23* and *4.24*.

Table 4.21: Diet as a related cause of illness and health problems

	Yes %	No %
Lung cancer	5.4	94.6
Arthritis	30.3	69.7
Heart disease	89.4	10.6
Diabetes	70.0	30.0
High blood pressure	84.6	15.4
Tonsillitis	0.8	99.2
Constipation	88.7	11.3
Obesity	95.8	4.2
Bowel cancer	53.5	46.5
Tooth decay	88.6	11.4
Gallbladder stones	46.5	53.5
Stomach cancer	50.4	49.6
Anaemia	61.8	38.2
Thalassaemia	4.8	95.2
Breast cancer	8.6	91.4
Cataracts	9.2	90.8

Of most significance, perhaps, in *Table 4.21* is the large proportion who were not aware of the link between diet and anaemia (38%) and diet and diabetes (30%).

Table 4.22: Alcohol as a contributory factor to health problems

	Yes %	No %
Anaemia	17.6	82.4
Car accidents	99.3	0.7
High blood pressure	86.4	13.6
AIDS	4.0	96.0
Lung cancer	14.0	86.0
Stomach ulcers	83.2	16.8
Chickenpox	0.0	100.0
Arthritis	9.5	90.5
Impotence	66.5	33.6
Liver cancer	97.9	2.1

The respondents seem to have a good knowledge about the health problems that are more likely to occur in people who drink alcohol. It was surprising to find that just over one third of respondents did not associate impotence with drinking, however this may be due to the over representation of women in the sample.

Table 4.23: Smoking as a contributory factor to health problems

	Yes %	No %
Heart attack	88.4	11.6
Bronchitis	93.2	6.8
Arthritis	16.4	83.6
High blood pressure	65.9	34.1
Stomach ulcer	55.1	44.9
Lung cancer	97.2	2.8
Diabetes	15.0	85.0
Stroke	62.8	37.2
Tonsillitis	29.5	70.5
Tooth decay	40.1	59.9

Around one third of respondents were not knowledgeable about the association between smoking and high blood pressure and stroke, whereas a majority were aware of the association with heart attack. This may reflect the emphasis of health promotion programmes on the effects of smoking on the heart and lungs.

Table 4.24: Stress as a contributory factor to health problems

	Yes %	No %
Heart attack	97.3	2.7
Bronchitis	12.9	87.1
Arthritis	12.9	87.1
High blood pressure	97.3	2.7
Stomach ulcer	87.1	12.9
Diabetes	29.1	70.9
Asthma	54.1	45.9
Tonsillitis	11.3	88.7
Headaches	98.7	1.3
Diarrhoea	51.9	48.1

Knowledge about the effects of stress on health was generally good.

Knowledge and health behaviour

In order to explore the relationship between knowledge (about diet, alcohol, smoking and stress), its effects on the diseases in the tables above and actual health behaviours, knowledge scores were constructed.

The findings revealed that eating and knowledge about diet were not correlated: almost equal proportions (around 50%) of those with a high knowledge score ate a poor diet as those who had a low knowledge score. Equal proportions of those with a high score on knowledge about the harmful effects of smoking were regular smokers as of those with a low score. A similar absence of association was also found between knowledge about the benefits of exercise and exercise participation, as already discussed in *Section 5*. These findings indicate that knowledge alone does not lead people to live healthier lifestyles.

Sexual health

Respondents were asked to report whether they had used condoms in the last year. Of the 111 who answered, over a quarter (27%) said they had; 11% said they regularly carry condoms to protect themselves from sexually transmitted diseases. They were then asked whether they would avoid using condoms for the reasons listed in *Table 4.25*.

Table 4.25: Sexual health: Reasons for avoiding the use of condoms

	Yes %	No %	Not sure %
Obtaining condoms is too embarrassing	9.2	82.7	8.2
Condoms are too expensive	6.3	76.0	17.7
There aren't enough machines when you need to buy some	6.3	64.6	29.2
I can't get condoms from my GP on perscription	3.2	64.9	31.9
Condoms reduce sensitivity	34.4	51.6	14.0
My partner would not like using condoms	21.7	63.0	15.2
You look cheap if you carry condoms	9.6	78.7	11.7

The main reason given for not using condoms was that they reduce sensitivity and secondly that they felt their partner would not like using them.

Discussion of findings

The findings in this section of my survey indicate that the Greek Cypriots have a fairly good knowledge of the factors that cause heart disease and of the effects of their behaviour on their health. However, there is an inconsistency between knowledge and behaviour. Respondents continue to follow unhealthy practice even when they indicated that they were aware of these. As mentioned earlier, knowledge alone does not lead to healthier lifestyles. Some of the responses to the statements about the respondents' beliefs about the onset of heart attacks indicates that individuals function within a 'fatalistic-realistic-idealist' health belief model which is sustained by a strong dose of denial. It is probably the denial that influences people's motivation and action. Bouri (1992) found that many of her informants explicitly denied the existence of illness in themselves and their families. This is not surprising if we consider that health is considered as a prerequisite for one's ability to function properly as a member of the society, meaning being productive. Being able to work hard and earn as much as one could was the philosophy that the first generation of migrants adopted, most of whom left Cyprus for a better economic future as discussed in *Chapter 1*. This philosophy is still very evident today. Often the type of work and pressure of work (working in restaurants, owning a shop or a small factory, doing piece-work, etc.) may be the cause of self neglect or adopting risky health behaviours. All these point towards the need for focusing on health promotion strategies that will aim at motivating the Greek Cypriots to look after their health.

Section 11: Finding out about health issues

Topics about which respondents would like to know more

Table 4.26 lists the participants' responses to a number of topics about which they wished to have more information.

Table 4.26: Topics about which the respondents would like more information

	Yes %	No %
Plans of local hospitals and community services for following year	72.4	27.6
Reduce risk of having a heart attack	72.1	27.9
Reduce stress in their life	70.3	29.7
Eating a healthier diet	68.1	31.9
Health Authority's plan for following year	64.9	34.2
Getting a better night's sleep	46.6	53.4
Losing weight	45.0	55.0
Reduce risk of getting HIV/AIDS	24.0	76.0
Giving up smoking	17.6	82.4
Cutting down on alcohol	9.9	90.1

Discussion of findings

During the last five to ten years enormous changes have happened to the national health service system. For those working within the system, the majority of these changes seem inevitable and desirable. Demographic, epidemiological, technological, economic and political forces are driving these changes. The *Health of the Nation* strategy (DoH, 1992) emphasised the importance of informing local people of any proposed changes and of involving them in planning and decision making. During the fieldwork which proceeded this survey and which was done during 1992–4, I discovered that Greek Cypriot people were very ignorant about the changes that were taking place or the general direction towards a primary care led NHS. They had heard of or witnessed hospital closures and they were very critical about this change. The majority saw the hospital as the focus of health care and their judgements about the NHS were totally hospital based; those who had had 'positive hospital experiences' tended to think that the NHS was marvellous while those who had encountered 'negative hospital experiences' thought that the NHS was going from bad to worse. It is interesting to note that by 1995 people were putting their wish to learn more about the health authority's plans on top of their list. This in my view indicates the failure of the Health Authority to inform and involve the local population in an effective way. This failure shows very clearly how difficult it is to change traditional ways of operating and, perhaps most importantly, of changing the ideology of 'the professionals know best' to one which requires a balance in this power relationship.

Reducing the risk of having a heart attack, eating a healthier diet and reducing stress, are all connected and reflect many of the previous findings in my study. Greek Cypriots are well aware of levels of heart disease within our community and its associated causes. The community fears heart disease because it affects young and old and because it can have sudden and devastating effects. However, during the last ten years the government has funded a number of initiatives which aimed at informing the public about these issues. In view of this topic featuring so prominently in the priorities of the Greek Cypriot community, as well as the evidence that this survey has provided, we need to question whether the message is getting through. The effectiveness of health education programmes in general is continuously being debated at national level. At a more local level, there must be more investment in finding the most effective and culturally sensitive methods of delivering such programmes to meet the needs of local communities. It is often assumed by health planners and providers that the only problem faced by the Greek Cypriot community is that of language related to individuals from the first generation. This is clearly wrong.

Section 12: Views

Of the 151 participants, 63 offered a range of views about how we could all work towards making the Greek Cypriot community in Enfield and Haringey healthier. Their views fall into the following categories:

* the need for information
* the need for education
* the need for services
* the need for Greek speaking staff
* other suggestions

The need for information

Respondents suggested the need for information at two levels: for adults and for children/teenagers. Most of them have indicated that the Greek community needs to be provided with information on healthy eating and exercise. Respondents were concerned that children/ teenagers should be provided with information regarding sexual health and the risks of HIV/AIDS as well as diet and exercise. It has been proposed that this information should be provided in the form of leaflets, available at both clinics and community centres and also regularly mailed to Greek people. The need for reinforcing this information at regular intervals was highlighted through the suggestion of the production of a newsletter on health topics. Many emphasised the use of Greek radio and newspapers as very appropriate media for the dissemination of such information.

The need for education

This is related to the need for information. Respondents suggested that the Greek community needs to be educated on the topics mentioned above through meetings with guest speakers who will provide the 'real facts' about these topics thus raising peoples' awareness and knowledge. It was recommended that cookery demonstrations could be used which would enable individuals to cook more healthily while maintaining the Greek traditions. Another topic highlighted for action was the need for 'stop smoking' programmes.Greek schools were seen as having an important role to play in educating children and young people towards healthier lifestyles. The need for a co-ordinated approach between Greek schools, Greek radio, Greek newspapers and Greek community organisations was also identified. This is an important indicator of the wish of the Greek community to initiate action and take control of their health.

The need for services

This was mainly around two areas: the need for nursing/old peoples homes with Greek speaking carers and the need for a Greek community centre. Many of the respondents appeared concerned about the growing number of elderly needing care, some of whom would eventually be unable to continue living at home. In view of their language difficulties (and it appears that of many others) it was repeatedly recommended that there is an urgent need for more Greek speaking staff and interpreters. The need for a Greek community centre was probably highlighted by those living in the London Borough of Enfield where such a centre does not exist, whereas these are provided in the London Borough of Haringey. Respondents viewed such centres as the focus for accessible and appropriate information, education and health promotion services including health check-ups and screening. Such centres were also viewed as meeting places for socialising, exchanging ideas and sharing problems as well as for recreational events encompassing keep-fit classes.

Other services that were featured are, more female doctors who would deal with gender related health problems, as according to one respondent, 'a lot of women would rather not have the examination done [cervical smear] if they can't be examined by a female doctor. For some this can be fatal', or as another respondent expressed it, 'trying to encourage women about the importance of having the various tests, like cervical smears, breast screening etc. which many still find embarrassing to come forward to have'.

The need for Greek speaking staff

Many respondents expressed concern about the dearth of Greek speaking health professionals such as doctors, nurses and carers. The rationale for this, as discussed above, was the number of first generation people who have language difficulties. More important than language is perhaps the ability to provide culturally sensitive and competent care; the respondents seem to imply that by having more members of the Greek community entering these professions they would not only provide such care themselves, but they would also help others to understand the Greek culture and apply this knowledge when caring for Greek people.

In addition to the above the need for more Greek interpreters was identified, especially for hospitals and GP surgeries.

Other suggestions

Is was suggested that the Greek community needs to be encouraged through various means to become more open about mental illness. As one respondent expressed it, 'The mentally ill need a lot more support and the community should stop seeing them as a shame to society.' Such comments imply that mental illness is still regarded as a stigma within the Greek community.

There was a plea that doctors should give more time to people in order to discuss their problems more fully. The issue of waiting times, both for GPs or a hospital appointment, was also raised.

Finally, a minority of respondents took a more passive or fatalistic view regarding the health of the Greek community, typically expressed by one respondent as, 'Leave it to the experts,' and another, 'The Greeks are pretty thick when it comes to these matters. I do not think that they will listen.'

Discussion of findings

The findings of this section confirm some of the findings in the previous sections but also serve to highlight the major concerns of the respondents. These findings strongly suggest the need for more information and education; most importantly they raise the issue of accessibility and appropriateness of such information and education. However, the sheer focus on these needs also highlights the lack of awareness of the respondents of the available information and health education. These negative findings need to be taken into account by those who plan and provide these services to ensure that messages are reaching those for whom they are intended and that resources are not unnecessarily wasted. One way of achieving this would be to increase the involvement of the Greek community and to adopt a collaborative model of service development and delivery, including the relevant local authority departments.

The concerns about diet and exercise were very appropriately identified as the most important health issues; this view is backed up by the findings of this survey as discussed in earlier sections.

In relation to the need for services the evidence points towards the development of a self-help culture within the Greek community. All the indicators signify that Greek people wish to be involved in their own health care and that of their community in general. They are concerned about the 'now' (their wish to have community centres) but are also planning for the future (provision of homes and services for the elderly). These concerns are in contrast to those expressed by some respondents who suggested that these issues are best left to the experts. We now see another aspect of the model that began emerging in section 10 'fatalistic-realistic-idealistic', this being the 'active-passive' dimension.

A lot was said about the need for Greek speaking health professionals. This issue deserves some comment for two inter-connected reasons. The first is that of Greek representation in health care professions. Anthias (1992) reported that Cypriots are under-represented in the professional occupations and over-represented in the self-employed and small employer category and in semi-skilled and unskilled work. This, she argues, is the result of the migration processes associated with Greek Cypriots, for example, the type of migrant, the reasons for migration, the cultural value system of migrants, as well as the difficulties and discrimination which they faced in this country. Their experiences had influenced and still do influence them and their families, resulting in many of their children underachieving at school, or being encouraged to work in family businesses. The situation is gradually changing and we are seeing a few second generation individuals taking up a career in medicine. This, however seems to be the exception. The Greek community, like many other communities, has always viewed medicine as one of the most noble professions. The same cannot be said about nursing or midwifery. Most Greek people greatly appreciate the care they receive from nurses and midwives but would not like their daughters and least of all their sons to enter these professions. The evidence I gathered during the group and individual interviews which I conducted in 1993, and during another small study on this topic which I conducted with a colleague in 1995–6, suggests that Greek Cypriots continue to hold the traditional negative views about these professions (Papadopoulos and Tilki, 1996).

This position illustrates another contradiction: Greek Cypriots recognise the need and value of having members of their community working as health care professionals but, despite this, they continue to discourage their children from entering the biggest caring professions.

Another area where attitudinal change is not occurring (or if it is, extremely slowly) is that of mental illness. This remains a stigma within the community; many families would not only not admit to having one of their members suffering from it, they would try to conceal it. As discussed in an earlier section, many individuals are reporting high levels of stress; the womens' study revealed that many of them suffer from mental health problems and some are on medication. But while 'suffering with my nerves' (the term usually used to express stress or depression) is very often openly shared with others who demonstrate sympathy and understanding having a family member suffering from schizophrenia or any other mental illness that requires hospitalisation or renders the individual less capable of having a 'normal life', would be associated with madness. It is no wonder that families often try to conceal it, often try to deal with the person without seeking help. Mental illness is an area which clearly needs to be opened up, discussed and dealt with.

Finally, the issue of long waiting times was again highlighted in the respondents' comments. Long waiting times for hospital treatments has been one of the government's target areas for improvement and some reductions are periodically reported in the annual 'league tables' published by the government (statistics on the performance of health services). This undoubtedly needs to be taken into consideration when discussing the Greek Cypriots' reports of waiting too long for a hospital appointment or (much more frequently reported) for a GP appointment. As discussed in a previous section, there is evidence to support the view that people from minority ethnic groups do not simply have a natural aversion to waiting, or that they expect to be seen on demand, but that they are experiencing indirect discrimination from racist staff and policies. This results in having to wait longer. But if certain community groups find – particularly when it comes to seeing the GP – it difficult to accept the appointment system, to insist on adhering to it, when it may be failing often large numbers of particular groups, would be unreasonable. The system, like any other system, needs to be under constant review and adjusted to suit the differing client groups.

References

Anthias F (1988) Aspects of ethnicity, class and generation among Greek Cypriots in Britain. In: Bouras N, Littlewood R eds. *Stress and Coping in the Greek Communities in Britain*. Research Evaluation and Development Unit, Division of Psychiatry, Guy's Hospital, London

Anthias F (1992) *Ethnicity, Class, Gender and Migration*. Avebury, Aldershot.

Bouri P (1992) *Gender, Ethnicity and Health Patterns: The attitudes of Greek Cypriot Women Towards Breast Cancer and Screening Programmes*. Unpublished MSc dissertation, Brunel University

Brown GW, Harris T (1979) *Social Origins of Depression*. Tavistock, London

Colhoun H, Prescott-Clark P (eds) (1996) *Health Survey for England*. Vols I and II. Social and Community Planning Research, Dept of Epidemiology and Public Health, University College, HMSO, London.

Constantinides P (1977) The Greek Cypriots: factors in the maintenance of ethnic identity. In: Watson JL ed. *Between Two Cultures. Migrants and Minorities in Britain*. Basil Blackwell, Oxford

Constantinides P (1988) Service provision. In: Bouras N, Littlewood R eds. *Stress and Coping in the Greek Communities in Britain*. Research Evaluation and Development Unit, Division of Psychiatry, Guy's Hospital, London

Department of Health (1992) *On the State of Public Health 1991*. HMSO, London

Department of Health (1992) *The Health of the Nation: a strategy for health in England*. HMSO, London

Department of Health and Social Security (1984) *Committee on Medical Aspects of Food Policy: Diet and Cardiovascular Disease.* HMSO, London

Department of Health (1995) *Variations in Health. What Can the Department of Health and the NHS Do?* HMSO, London

Department of Statistics and Research, Ministry of Finance (1993) *Health and Hospital statistics 1991* Series I, report No. 12. (ISSN 0258 - 7955) Republic of Cyprus, Nicosia

Fernando S (1991) *Mental Health, Race and Culture.* Macmillan and Mind Publications, London

Folkman S, Lazrus RS (1988) The relationship between coping and emotion: Implications for theory and research. *Soc Sci and Med* **26**(3): 309–17

George V, Millerson G (1967) The Cypriot community in London. *Race,* **8**:77–92

Harrington B *et al* (1993) *Health and lifestyles in Newcastle: The Newcastle Health and Lifestyle Survey 1991.* Dept of Public Health Medicine, Newcastle Health Authority and Dept of Epidemiology and Public Health, University of Newcastle

Health Education Authority (1991) *Enjoy Healthy Eating.* HEA, London

Health Education Authority (1994) *Health and Lifestyles. Black and Minority Ethnic Groups in England.* HEA, London

Helman CG (1990) *Culture, Health and Illness 2nd edtion.* Butterworth Heineman, Oxford

Report on the work of the Department of Medical Services and Public Health (1995). Republic of Cyprus, Nicosia

Kiritz S, Moos RH (1974) Physiological effects of social environment. *Psychosom Med* **36**:96–113

Littlewood R (1988) Ethnic minorities and mental health in Britain: an overview, with some hypotheses for the Greek communities. In: Bouras N, Littlewood R eds. *Stress and Coping in the Greek Communities in Britain.* Evaluation and Development Unit, Diviosion of Psychiatry, Guy's Hospital, London

London Borough of Enfield (1993) *1991 Census. Summary paper No:3. Ethnic minorities.* LBE, London

McNaught A (1987) *Health Action and Ethnic Minorites.* National Community Health Resource and Bedford Square Press, London

Nabarro JDN (1988) Diabetes in the United Kingdom: some facts and figures. *Diabetic Medicine* **5**:816–22

New River Health Authority (1993) *New River Sector Profiles.* London

Oakley R (1970) The Cypriots in Britain. *Race Today* **2**:99–102

Oakley R (1987) *Changing Patterns of Distribution of Cypriot Settlements.* Centre for Research in Ethnic Relations. Research papers in Ethnic Relations No5. University of Warwick

Papadopoulos I, Worrall L (1996) *All Health Care is Good until you have a Problem: An Examination of the Primary Health Care Needs of the Greek and Greek Cypriot Women.* Greek and Greek Cypriot Women of Enfield, London

Papadopoulos I, Tilki M (1996) *Not for us. The Cypriots' Views About Nursing and Midwifery.* A report for the community liaison committee. Middlesex University

Tokas N (1995) 2000 die from heart disease. *Parikiaki* August 10th, p 5

Royal College of Physicians (1991) Medical aspects of exercise: benefits and risks. *J RColl Physicians Lond* **25**:193–6

Steinberg H, Sykes EA (1993) Mood enhancement throughhysical exercise-Introduction to workshop on health, sport and physical exercise. In: Schroder H ed. *Health Psychology. Potential in diversity.* S. Roderer Verlag, Regensburg

Storkey M (1994) *London's Ethnic Minorities. One City Many Communities. An Analysis of 1991 Census Results.* London Research Centre, London

Theodorou Z (1992) *Alcohol and the Invisible Communities. Needs and Attitudes in the Cypriot and Turkish Groups.* Haringey Advisory Group on Alcohol, London

The Sports Council and the Health Education Authority (1992) *Allied Dunbar National Fitness Survey, Summary Report.* HEA and Sports Council, London

Weinman J (1981) *An Outline of Psychology as Applied to Medicine.* Wright, Bristol

White A *et al* (1993) *Health Survey for England 1991.* OPCS. HMSO, London

5

The health of the Irish in Britain

Mary Tilki

The Irish have migrated to Britain for centuries and, while there has been a considerable body of historical material, there has been little attention from a sociological perspective until relatively recently (Williams, 1992). This recognition has stemmed from a few researchers and voluntary groups predominantly from within the Irish community in Britain and almost certainly borne out of concern for a disadvantaged group. Agencies in Britain concerned with issues of ethnicity and discrimination have persistently ignored the existence of the Irish, classifying them with the indigenous population or a host of other white minorities such as the Poles or the Cypriots. In recent years the Irish have been described variously as 'a race apart' (O' Meachair, 1992) or 'an invisible minority' (Pearson *et al*, 1991).

Although some differences exist, the social and health problems of Irish people are similar to those experienced by other minority groups. However, the tendency to view ethnicity in terms of black skin colour, with or without language differences means that Irish people have not to date been considered a minority ethnic group. Many Irish people themselves are uncomfortable with the idea and are reluctant to identify with the negative images of minorities that pervade British society. The stereotype of the drunken, stupid Paddy or the terrorist is not an attractive image to aspire to, whether one has achieved success or is struggling to survive. Connor (1987) suggests that there is a tendency among Irish people to keep a low profile and to opt for 'a kind of invisibility, merging into the host community as far as possible.' There has also been a corresponding tendency for researchers to overlook the Irish or to treat them as part of the British population. That is not to say that monitoring of the Irish community has not taken place, but it has largely served other purposes and in particular security needs (Greenslade *et al*, 1991). However, the ceasefire in Northern Ireland and media publicity around Irish dancing and music have seen an emergence of pride in being Irish by many well-known figures and ordinary Irish people. There is an increasing current of interest among researchers, students and academics and an expanding body of interesting but worrying material is emerging.

The invisible Irish

At a social policy or political level it is all too easy to equate whiteness with homogeneity and neglect any examination of the experiences of Irish (or other white) people. It could be argued that the state has directed minority group demands into competition, with each group having to prove its disadvantage in a hierarchy of oppression. In addition, ideas of assimilation and uniformity serve to mask ethnic differences. Colour has become a marker of belonging; being of the same colour as the host community suggests being of the same nation, which implies no possibility of discrimination (Hickman and Walter, 1995).Whatever factors or combination of factors make the Irish invisible the outcome of statistical invisibility is political invisibility (Ni Bhrolochain, 1990). Ethnicity data are needed to document discrimination and disadvantage, to plan action to remedy these and to evaluate the effectiveness of adopted policies. It is salutary to remember that evidence alone cannot combat disadvantage. Political will is crucial, and it is only within this context that data can be useful. Despite problems with ethnicity data there has been evidence of multiple disadvantage among Irish people for many years (Connor, 1987; Burke, 1976; Burns and O'Meaehair, 1988.) but prevarication and resistance from state bodies means that it has been addressed with reluctance and only in a limited way.

A profile of the Irish community in Britain

There are difficulties with statistical evidence in relation to the Irish in Britain. The practice of counting by country of birth until 1991 meant that only those who were born in Ireland were included in data. Those who were born in Britain of Irish parents and those women married to heads of household who were not Irish were excluded. The 1991 census was the first to include an ethnicity category but there was no classification specifically for Irish people except under 'any other ethnic group'. Despite these difficulties it is clear that there are some 837,500 Irish born people in Britain forming 1.5% of the population. It is also suggested that about 3.5% of the population is living in a household where the head or the partner of the household head is Irish. The age structure of the Irish born community in Britain is different from that of other minority groups and the white population as a whole. It is a significantly older population with many in the post–retirement group and a large proportion in the pre- pension age cohort. As with the host society there is a greater number of women in the older age bands, in particular women who were born in the Republic of Ireland.

Table 5.1: People born in Ireland compared with white people and people from minority ethnic groups

Age group	White %	Ethnic Minority group %	Born in Northern Ireland %	Born in Republic of Ireland %
0–4	6.35	11.1	1.2	0.6
5–15	13.0	22.0	4.65	2.75
16–24	12.5	16.4	9.25	5.0
25–44	28.0	32.5	34.0	27.0
45–59/64	19.7	14.5	27.8	37.85
60/65+	19.35	4.4	20.1	26.65

Adapted from Owen (1995) Table 1. Statistical paper 9

There are also significant differences in marital status among Irish people Older women and particularly men are statistically more likely never to have married. Employment patterns in earlier life which meant low and often irregular pay and required geographic mobility gave few opportunities to find partners and settle down. The older age span of the cohort means that many, especially the women, are widowed. Perhaps the most surprising of all is the high incidence of divorce – almost double the rate of the white population and other minority groups (Owen, 1995). The higher tendency to be alone in adulthood or in old age has major implications for social and health services due to the absence of family support networks.

Patterns of migration

Irish people have left Ireland in waves of emigration since the Great Famine of the 1840s. As with other colonised countries, Ireland had nothing to offer particular sections of the community because of the systematic underdevelopment of the Irish economy by Britain (Crotty, 1986). In addition land customs preventing the division of land into small units meant that only one family member could inherit. Since this invariably meant the eldest son, other children had little choice but to emigrate. It has been argued that while there was little to offer economically, many still saw emigration as an opportunity not to be missed (Ryan, 1990). This 'pull' factor was fuelled by letters from abroad citing high wages, abundant work opportunities and frequently enclosing the cost of the fare (Brody, 1973). The effect was magnified by the loneliness and isolation experienced by young people whose friends had all gone away leaving them with few opportunities for youthful social activity. Similar to people from the West Indies mentioned in *Chapter 3*, emigration was a fact of life for Irish people. For most the place of choice was America, but the restricted immigration of the 1920s and the depression of the 1930s meant reduced migration to America. The cost of the fare to America was prohibitive unless provided by family already abroad. The only alternative for most was Britain, and emigrants generally went there reluctantly. It is important to remember that emigration was not a choice that was taken willingly by the majority but was forced of necessity. This was evident by the slow pace of migration and the large numbers returning to Ireland in the boom years of the 1970s (Greenslade *et al,* 1991).

The experience of migration is recorded in a wealth of Irish literature in Gaelic, and more commonly English, and in the traditional and modern music that is the backbone of Irish culture. Literature and song in the past have tended to emphasise the grief of those leaving and of those left behind. In more recent times there has been some recognition of the difficulties faced by Irish people in their new lives such as the disaffection described in Christy Moore's song 'Picadilly's Neon Lights' or Dolores Keane' s 'Nothing to show for it all'. It is ironic however that there is little acknowledgement in Ireland of the sadness and the difficulties experienced by those who left their native soil throughout its history. It is still perceived that to leave was an easier option than to stay. Such denial is manifest in language which refers to migration rather than emigration and mobility rather than diaspora. It is also seen in the belief that Irish migrants are now among the highly educated and most successful in Europe, without recognition that a significant number of those who leave are neither educated nor skilled (Hickman and Walter, 1997).

Records indicate that emigration was essential for the survival of the family at home (Brody, 1973). However, the contribution of those who left home is usually forgotten. In 1958 a conservative estimate suggested that income from family members abroad constituted 2.5 % of national income and between 1958 and 1964, although the percentage fell slightly, the remittances were calculated at some 13 million pounds. Women in particular made regular if small payments to the upkeep of the family, whereas from men payments were higher but more sporadic (Brody, 1973). The need to make remittances to the family, coupled with low pay or sporadic employment, left many Irish women and men little income for their own use or to provide for themselves in the future. It is rarely noted that the exodus of large numbers from an area meant better chances for those who remained. (Ryan, 1990)

Gender and migration

It is important to distinguish a particular pattern of migration when considering Irish people because gender patterns differ between the Irish and other migrant groups. The significant difference is in the high incidence of women migrating alone, a pattern which has not occurred in any other community. It is argued, that although the primary reasons for leaving were economic , additional factors played a part in women's migration (O'Carroll, 1990). Since only the eldest son could inherit the land there were few prospects or choices for the women in the family. Marriage was an option provided there was an adequate dowry to make a woman an attractive proposition to a man and his family. Marriages were frequently arranged on the basis of wealth rather than love and young women were often matched to men who were considerably older than they were. Such arrangements are well recorded in poetry, song and in oral history. Marriage was not an easy life, as a woman was likely to be pregnant or nursing a child for most of her reproductive years while also working on the farm, milking, harvesting and keeping house. Although marriage did carry social status women got scant reward for their contribution and even the money earned from selling eggs, milk or chickens belonged to the husband. The social stigma of remaining single was worse for many than an arranged marriage. If a woman chose to remain single she would be required to work the farm and in the home as well as being scorned for being 'on the shelf'. One alternative for women was the religious life; this offered status and security, and vows of poverty chastity and obedience were probably no more harsh than life as a single or married woman. Training as a nurse or teacher were open to educated young women but since they had to be paid for they were only available to those who could afford them. Domestic service was open to some but the work was hard and the women exploited. The only alternative for many Irish women was emigration. Unlike women from other minorities they left home at a young age and alone to seek opportunities for advancement and for some to escape the oppression of a patriarchal society. Domestic service was the main source of employment for Irish women until the outbreak of the Second World War after which they were actively recruited for munitions factories and especially as nurses. The offer of accommodation was attractive and ensured a measure of security. Those who were not recruited to specific jobs usually stayed with friends or family until a job and accommodation was found.

Heterogeneity and Irish people

The Irish, like any other ethnic community, are not a single homogeneous group. As many differences can be found within them as can be found between them and other cultural groups. Irish people may have been born in the Irish Republic or in Northern Ireland and reflect the different cultural and religious traditions of either community. The two main religions in Northern Ireland are Prodestant and Catholic, a difference which has been the cause of much grief in Ireland's history. People born in the Irish Republic are more likely to be Catholics, and while some may not practice their religion it is an important factor in their cultural identity and has shaped their experience and their attitudes. It is argued that the Catholic Church has had a major influence on the state and has served to perpetuate orthodox attitudes to issues like divorce, contraception and abortion (Rossiter, 1993). Although there is much evidence that times are changing older people are still likely to retain old values.

Irish people come from both rural and urban areas and therefore have different experiences in terms of education and employment. Older people are more likely to have originated from rural communities and migrated as unskilled workers. Most older women particularly, as girls would have had an elementary education but were otherwise unprepared for migration. In the 1950s and 1960s a similar trend continued, but Irish women who were better educated than their male contemporaries were actively recruited to train as nurses providing a dedicated and respected workforce for the developing National Health Service. In the 1970s people began to return to Ireland to a booming economy. However the boom was shortlived and in the 1980s a new pattern of emigration emerged. This time those who left were educated, often to degree level, and were to find employment in a different sector of the economy from their earlier counterparts. Despite the persistence of the 'stupid' stereotype it is clear that a large percentage of Irish people , particularly those from Northern Ireland, are highly qualified. It is evident that many Irish people are successful but it is easy to forget the considerable numbers who are less fortunate.

Employment patterns

Irish people have high participation rates in the labour market. Although there are greater numbers in the retired bracket, economic activity is similar to that of white people and better than most minority groups (Owen, 1995). Irish people are to be found across all occupational groups with concentrations in particular areas of the workforce depending on gender and whether born in the Republic of Ireland or Northern Ireland. People from Northern Ireland are significantly more likely to be in white-collar jobs. Men born in Northern Ireland are more likely to be in white collar jobs while men from the Republic of Ireland work mainly in the as labourers or other less skilled occupations. Women from both parts of Ireland are the backbone of the British nursing workforce and as such may be classified in a different socio-economic group than their male counterparts. Irish women are more likely to withdraw from the paid labour market while raising a family and not register as unemployed. Unemployment rates vary and analysis by industry indicates that unemployment levels are highest in the construction industry. Low income from low paid or sporadic employment undoubtedly plays an important role in patterns of health and housing and augments the deleterious effects of occupation

Housing status

Although there is a tremendous variation in economic activity among Irish people, significant numbers are in receipt of low income. Irish people are more likely to be living in the public and private rented sectors than in owner– occupation. They are significantly more likely to be in poor quality accommodation, sharing amenities, overcrowded and without central heating. Irish people make up to 50% of those making use of night shelters and other services for street homeless people. They are less likely to own consumer durables that the rest of the white population enjoy (Owen, 1995). Today young Irish women follow the same patterns as their predecessors, but fewer employment opportunities, increased rent costs and various types of harassment force them to them to move frequently with subsequent impact on their well-being (Cara, 1995). There are a number of concerns about older workers who, because of illness, redundancy or retirement, are evicted from tied accommodation rendering them homeless. The high level of long-term disability in the Irish community suggests that many are likely to be living in accommodation inappropriate for their needs.

Occupational injury

Rarely a week goes by without the Irish newspapers in Britain reporting a death or serious injury resulting from faulty equipment or inadequate safety provision on a construction site. Britain's record on building site safety has been raised at the United Nations Committee on Human Rights by the human rights watchdog Liberty as well as the Institute of

Employment Rights. In addition to a high incidence of fatality and serious injury the nature of work in which a large proportion of Irish men are employed gives rise to an increased level of occupational illness. Further research is needed, but evidence from front line agencies indicates that disability may be manifest at an earlier age than in the host community or other minority groups. Evidence from front line agencies suggests that men in particular experience high levels of musculoskeletal disorders like rheumatism and arthritis in their late forties or early fifties. This probably reflects heavy labour like lifting and digging and working in inclement weather as well as a high incidence of occupational injuries. At present there are particular concerns about a necrotic bone condition which affects former tunnel workers, a large proportion of whom are from three counties in Ireland. It would also be interesting to explore the incidence of deafness in construction workers who were not provided with or chose not to use safety equipment to protect hearing. A large proportion of men who are economically inactive are permanently sick. This may reflect the high incidence of industrial injuries, or it may indicate older men moving from long-term unemployment to sickness benefit (Owen, 1995). The incidence of back injury in nurses is also high and since nursing is a major source of occupation for Irish women it is easy to imagine that some of the incapacity experienced in later life is related to the demands of the job and an environment where little attention was paid to safety until recently.

Social networks

The effects of disabling illness in Irish people is augmented by social factors such as housing status, income and social networks. The need to move from place to place for work meant that many Irish people, especially men, never set down roots. Coupled with low or sporadic income and the need to support the family in Ireland a large proportion of Irish people, particularly men, never married and are therefore more prone to be socially isolated in illness or in old age. The incidence of divorce and widowhood is higher than in the white community or in other minority ethnic groups and suggests a possible absence of support in times of family crisis or illness. Hundreds of Irish people die each year without the comfort or support of friends or family (Irish Post,

1994). A week rarely passes without an account of an Irish person whose death remains undetected for weeks or even months. Evidence from Irish community agencies highlight the isolation and loneliness experienced by many older Irish people.

Health patterns

While there are significant statistical problems, the available evidence demonstrates very clearly that the health of Irish people is poor in comparison with the indigenous population and most other minority groups (Balarajan and Bulusu, 1990). It is also consistently worse than that of the Irish in Ireland (Marmot *et al,* 1984; Kelleher and Hillier, 1996). The Irish population in Britain is an ageing one with a high proportion of members in the retired age group and a large number in the pre-retirement ageband. The age of the population in part contributes to the high levels of long term disability experienced by Irish people, but even controlling for age, the illness rates for Irish born people is still five to ten per cent higher than that of the host population (Owen, 1995). Irish people living in Britain have significantly higher mortality rates for a range of illnesses across all diagnostic categories, (Balarajan and Bulusu, 1990), and there is evidence that such patterns are continued into the second generation of Irish people (Raftery *et al,* 1990; Harding and Balarajan, 1996). Irish men in particular demonstrate considerable evidence of premature mortality for all diagnoses and a significant number die up to ten years earlier than their fellow countrymen who remained in Ireland (Marmot *et al,* 1984). It is also argued that improvements are fewer than in most other groups.

Theories of health

Various theoretical explanations have been offered over time to attempt to explain the poor health of the Irish in Britain. Explanations based on ideas of heredity are challenged by the lower mortality rates experienced by the population in Ireland (Williams, 1992). Social selection has been proposed as an explanation by several writers (Marmot *et al*, 1984; Raftery *et al*, 1990; Williams, 1992). It is argued that both positive and negative selection mechanisms can explain the health status of the Irish. Negative selection theories suggest that when people are ill and unable to work their economic position declines and they are forced to migrate. It is argued that in contrast to other groups the Irish had few barriers to entry and the less privileged were more likely to migrate. Should this be the case the expectation would be that over time migrant mortality would return to the level common to both England and Ireland. However, this is not borne out by studies into second generation Irish people (Raftery *et al,* 1990; Harding and Balarajan, 1996). With the exception of the daughters whose mother alone was born in Ireland, high mortality persists into the second generation (Raftery *et al,* 1990). Positive selection might explain migration from some parts of the world where only the fittest, economically and as regards health, are granted entry and may explain the improved mortality of second generation Irish women whose mothers appear to experience more rapid social mobility than men. This probably reflects educational and occupational qualifications or their mobility through marriage (Hornsby-Smith, 1987). The stress of migration is also proposed as an explanation for poor health in migrants. An extensive psychological literature exists on migration stress and culture shock especially when the new country is dissimilar from the home country (Furnham and Bockner, 1986; Oberg, 1954). Although there has been little attention to the experience of Irish people, oral history accounts in recent years throw some light on the challenges faced by Irish women (Lennon *et al,* 1988; O'Carroll, 1990). It might be expected that the ability to speak English, a fair skin and familiarity with a western lifestyle could enable Irish people to adjust more rapidly than migrants from far away parts of the world. It would appear that this superficial similarity may be more of a hindrance than a help. On migration the individual is confronted by his or her own identity and is reminded of the differences that exist between him/her and individuals in the new environment. (Kelleher and Hillier, 1996). Adapting to and accepting the inevitability of these differences high-lights the distance between old and new. Enforced migration and culture shock play a part in migration stress. However, it is difficult to isolate migration effects and cultural bereavement and it is probable that other factors are involved.

It could be argued that the poor health of Irish people is a feature of their low class position and that high rates of illness are to be expected of such a group. Poorer economic circumstances, and the working conditions common to manual workers, may well contribute to the relatively poor health of Irish people in Britain. However even in Social Class 1 the SMR was significantly higher than for English men aged 15–64 (Marmot *et al,* 1984). This suggests some other factor, and in the absence of a clear genetic link, the focus has been on lifestyle and behaviour (Adelstein *et al,* 1986a). The incidence of smoking, alcohol consumption and access to health care have all been blamed for ill health in the Irish community. However there has been much less attention to structural factors, issues of ethnic identity and anti-Irish racism which may contribute to distress and cause ill health. Harding and Balarjan (1996) examined the causes of mortality and the influence of socio-economic factors on the mortality of second generation Irish people over a 19 year period and concluded that, despite some structural assimilation, entrenched economic and cultural differences in life chances still existed. Low income, sporadic employment and poor housing take their toll on health. Kelleher and Hillier (1996) considered issues of identity and suggested that the behaviour of Irish people both in Ireland and England is shaped by the history of Ireland and its relationship with England. Greenslade, drawing from the work of Fanon (1967), suggests that colonised people and their way of life is seen as inferior (1992). Irish people are protected until they emigrate but when exposed to stereotypical images of themselves as stupid or drunken are faced with the decision either to challenge or to ignore them. Either way results in tension and makes for difficulty in establishing a sense of identity. Anti-Irish racism still exists; to date case law is limited and largely ignored. However McCluskey (1989) argued that a significant proportion of Irish people believe that health is largely a matter of external control and not within their own sphere of influence. This he suggests relates to the experience of the Catholic faith and being socialised into a traditional and unquestioning society. This explanation is a popular one among Irish professionals but needs further exploration and analysis. Another often forgotten factor is the ambivalent attitudes to emigration held by those in Ireland, where some who leave are seen as traitors and others are given their blessing and seen as a way of preserving Ireland as a traditional and holy place (Ryan, 1990).

Given the stresses associated with identity, disadvantage and discrimination it is hardly surprising that Irish people resort to tobacco and alcohol use. What is clear is that no single perspective can explain the poor health status of Irish people in Britain. It is incumbent on all health professionals, and I would argue Irish professionals in particular, to challenge everyday assumptions and question the conventional wisdom of biomedical approaches to care.

Respiratory problems

Chronic obstructive airways diseases, such as chronic bronchitis, asthma and emphysema, attract little attention from researchers despite being major causes of disability in British society; it would appear that they are significantly higher in Irish people (Balarajan and Bulusu, 1990). At first sight it would appear that the high incidence of smoking among Irish men and women is the key (Balarajan and Yuen, 1986). There is little doubt that these disorders (as well as cancers) are related to tobacco smoking but there has been scant attention to wider socio-economic factors like poverty, poor housing and low income. Evidence suggests that cold, dampness and overcrowding contribute to respiratory disorders (Lowry, 1991). The poverty, poor housing and overcrowding which occur more frequently for Irish people (O'Meachair, 1992; Cara, 1994) undoubtedly account for the excessive mortality from tuberculosis in Irish people (Balarajan and Bulusu, 1990). Measures to improve respiratory health can only be effective if they take account of the wider social factors and aim to improve income and quality of life.

Coronary heart disease

Coronary heart disease is a major killer of our time. Its incidence in Irish people by Britain is surpassed only in the Asian community. The work of Raftery *et al* (1990) highlights its persistence into the second generation of Irish in Britain; there is little to suggest that trends are improving. Although mortality rates are highlighted it is highly probable that heart disease of a more chronic nature accounts for much of the disabling illness experienced by the Irish in England. The aetiology of coronary heart disease is complex but it could be argued that smoking and diet have a major role to play. *Health of the Nation* strategies include targets towards the reduction of smoking: if they are to be successful in the Irish community they need to adopt culturally sensitive approaches that recognise culturally conditioned attitudes to smoking in the Irish community. In a small study of Irish women it was evident that they were acutely aware of the relationship between smoking (and other factors) and health (Cara, 1995) but had little control over stressful aspects of their lives. Effective health promotion requires a recognition of structural factors which may lead people to smoke. Given the acceptability of smoking among many Irish people it could be argued that what is needed is an attitudinal social shift where it is increasingly unacceptable to smoke. Such changes must be directed specifically at the Irish community as a whole and be promoted by Irish professionals and agencies and initiated in places where Irish people gather.

Cancers

Research on the incidence of cancer points to an excess mortality due to most types of cancer in Irish people but in particular lung, lip, mouth and pharynx malignancies (Balarajan and Bulusu, 1990). This pattern differs from the indigenous population and especially from other minority groups where cancers are rarer. Few studies have examined exposure to cancer risk factors in minority groups, but trade unions in the construction industry are currently raising concern about asbestos. Given the nature of Irish men's work in the construction industry it is not difficult to imagine exposure to asbestos or other toxic irritants. The worldwide increase in skin cancer is also significant for the fair-skinned Irish who burn at the first sight of the sun. This is particularly important for Irish men whose role in the building trade exposes them to the sun in summer. The discomfort of physical work in the heat and possibly a certain macho culture leads them to remove their shirts and risk the dangers of burning thus increasing their risk of skin cancer.

Alcohol-related illness

Stereotypes of Irish people invariably include reference to alcohol and drunkenness. The reluctance to reinforce stereotypes has led to silen on the subject but it is important to challenge the myths while still recognising that problems do exist. Ireland has a high proportion of total abstainers but men who do drink tend to drink at high-risk levels in a pattern similar to high-consuming men in Yorkshire and Humberside (Harrison and Carr-Hill, 1992). Women are more likely to be abstainers but are no more likely to drink at high-risk levels than English or Welsh women. However it is acknowledged that a number of Irish people do suffer from alcohol related illness that seriously affects their physical mental and social health. Admissions for alcohol-related problems are up to seven times more common in Irish born people, especially in men. While there is some possibility of inappropriate diagnostic labelling in relation to alcoholism, the extent of the problem is a cause for concern. Harrison's work identifies very clearly that alcohol problems relate to transient housing, low income and social and relationship difficulties, but it is important to note that for the majority these problems occurred after leaving Ireland (Harrison and Carr-Hill, 1992). This evidence certainly challenges the negative selection hypothesis.

Despite research that clearly challenges the myth of the drunken Irish, there is still a tendency to assume that most illnesses are alcohol-related. Stomach ulcers and cancer may well remain undiagnosed in one who admits to a drinking habit. The low incidence of diabetes in Irish people may also reflect a neglect of thorough investigation if alcohol-related illness is suspected. Mortality from cirrhosis of the liver is significantly higher among Irish men than among other groups and it continues to rise. This rise is not exclusive to Irish people and is possibly related to the economic conditions of the last decade. This increased mortality may well be a reflection of health reforms guided more by financial than clinical judgements where decisions are made not to treat those who have contributed to their own illness. It may also be a product of the augmenting effects of poor nutrition and disadvantage which precipitate liver damage at fairly low levels of alcohol use.

Alcohol misuse is presented as a lifestyle factor for Irish people but, while evidence clearly demonstrates that most drinking problems occurred after leaving Ireland, there is no recognition of the wider social and psychological reasons why some Irish people drink to excess (Harrison and Carr-Hill, 1992). *Health of the Nation* targets can only realistically be achieved through a recognition of the pressures that lead

suse. Harrison and Carr-Hill demonstrate that Irish men
are reluctant to use statutory and non-statutory services
ose who do find Irish welfare agencies helpful and
There is obviously a need for specific service provision for
tho‿ alcohol problems which recognises and values the Irishness
of the individual and offers supportive and non-judgmental therapy. In
addition to the special skills of alcohol work, staff working in the field
need training in awareness of the nuances and conventions of Irish
culture. It is important that services 'reach out' to a group of people who
have low self-esteem and a considerable degree of peer pressure to
continue to drink. Outreach services can not only encourage people to
choose to seek help but can support them as they endeavour to change
lifestyle either by stopping drinking or by taking action to reduce harm.

Access to health care

It is easy for health and welfare professionals to blame the victim for
ill-health caused by smoking or other behaviours; it is particularly easy
when the individual colludes with the notion and willingly absorbs the
guilt. Irish people must be encouraged to have higher expectations of
health services, to realise they do not have to suffer in silence and that
they are entitled to help as a right. Although research in the area of
access is limited, what is available suggests that there is a high use of
acute services by people from minority groups. There is also some
suggestion that Irish people are reluctant to use health services until
forced to do so when their health has deteriorated. Irish people appeared
reluctant to consult on a range of health problems such as
musculoskeletal, urinary and ill-defined conditions although
consultation rates were high for respiratory disorders. They were also
less likely to be given a follow-up appointment and were less likely to
be visited at home (Gillam *et al*, 1989). These patterns of access conflict
with evidence of poor health and suggest low expectations of health and
health care but they may also suggest insensitive and ethnocentric
attitudes to Irish service users. The fear, and in some cases the reality, of
reproach prevents some individuals from seeking help. Personal and
professional attitudes contribute towards failure to seek or delay in
seeking health care. The individualisation of blame by either the
professional or the client deflects attention from structural factors that

cause unhealthy lifestyles or result in maladaptive coping strategies. There is limited research evidence (Harrison and Carr-Hill, 1992), but increasing anecdotal information from front-line Irish agencies, that culturally sensitive services are more likely to be used and valued.

HIV/AIDS

HIV and AIDS have a high prevalence in communities who have been marginalised from health and other social services. Therefore data is difficult to obtain but it is evident that the epidemiology of HIV/AIDs differs between Britain and Ireland. Compared to those in Britain the numbers are not only smaller but the mode of transmission is different. Ireland has a higher proportion of people diagnosed as infected by HIV or having AIDS who give drug use as the route of transmission. Ireland is also thought to have a higher rate of women who are HIV positive. Drug use is widespread in some of Ireland's larger cities; in certain parts of Dublin several members of one family may be affected by HIV or AIDS. The absence of drugs or HIV services in Ireland, and the stigma of either or both, means many leave home to seek access to health or other services in Britain (PIAA,1995).

Irish people who are gay often have difficulties with sexual identity in Ireland and leave home as a result. Puritanical attitudes to sexuality mean that safe sex may not be considered let alone negotiated. Irish people suffering from the health problems that are a part of AIDS are often alone and afraid. The first knowledge the family may be given is in severe illness or in the terminal stages. It is not easy for an ageing couple from a small country town to come to terms with their child's severe illness as well as their use of drugs or their homosexuality.

The Irish agency Positively Irish Action on AIDS (PIAA) helped prepare and support families shocked by being propelled into uncomfortable realities about their relatives in a big strange city. They provided information, advocacy and support to families caring for a person with AIDs and they helped the clients and families arrange transfer of care back to Ireland. Sadly this organisation was decommissioned by London healthcare purchasing consortia in1996 as it was believed that mainstream services could provide culturally sensitive care. To date there has been little evidence of culturally sensitive provision within the region. Evidence of unwillingness to use other services, and specific cultural needs, suggest a need for such provision.

Travellers

Irish travellers form a large proportion of the travelling population in Britain and tend to be drawn to London and other inner cities. They have a long and varied history in Ireland and can be traced back to pre-Christian times. Irish travellers originate from an itinerant tradespeople who moved from place to place working the harvest, trading horses and mending pots and pans. This explains the term 'tinker' which although once acceptable is now considered derogatory. The mechanisation of agriculture has made much of the traditional work carried out by travelling communities obsolete. The widespread use of plastic and enamel has reduced the demand for tinware and repairs. Changes in shopping habits and the increased use of cars has eliminated the need for household goods and trinkets formerly sold by travelling women. These changes have led to widespread migration into towns and cities where travellers have met economic and social marginalisation. Irish travellers have been exposed to hostility, discrimination and disadvantage at all levels of British society. They are frequently harassed by the police and neighbours. Despite protection under the race relations acts, other legislation related to town and country planning, highways and caravan sites has restricted travellers ability to lead a nomadic existence (LIWC, 1995). The failure to provide official sites and or to ensure provision of specific educational, social or medical support for travellers has an impact on the lives of travelling communities.

Discrimination against travellers continues to be tolerated despite race relations legislation and articles in the European Convention of Human Rights and United Nations International Covenant on Civil and Political Rights. Traveller site provision falls well short of demand. Travellers pay rent and council tax but get very little in return and have little security. There is an urgent need for statutory bodies and policy makers to recognise and respect the rights of travellers and to ensure that this minority are allowed to continue their long-shared history and cultural identity without persecution (LIWC, 1995). There is limited research on the health of Irish travellers, but studies of travellers in general broadly mirror the picture for other Irish people living in Britain. The health status of travelling people is significantly poorer than the norm. The incidence of stillbirth is 17 times higher than the national average and 12 times higher than among women in Social Class 5. Infant mortality is five times higher than the average and twice as many fall into the low birth weight category (Linthwaite, 1993). There is also a low uptake of ante-natal care, family planning, immunisation and developmental screening (Pahl and Vaile, 1986). Many travelling women are likely to be evicted in the late stages of pregnancy or in the early days after childbirth (Durward, 1990). It is argued that eviction around this time can have life-threatening effects for the women concerned and can also affect their long-term physical and mental health (Sadler, 1993).

It is also believed that there is a high incidence of congenital malformation among the children of travelling families (Linthwaite, 1993). It is usually assumed that this relates to consangunity, and the relationship to social, economic and environmental conditions remains unexplored. Accidents, burns and scalds are more common. Even on official campsites sanitation is inadequate thus predisposing children in particular to illness and infection (Vernon, 1994). Education for travelling children can be problematic whether they move frequently or are relatively settled. When families move about there is little continuity and even when fairly settled children go to school they are exposed to hostility and resentment. This compounds their unwillingness to attend school and results in low levels of literacy which in turn impairs access to health and welfare services. Male life expectancy is lower and premature death from circulatory disease is more common than even in the lowest socio-economic groups in the host population (Crout, 1987; Wilson, 1988). Smoking is also more common and women in particular suffer from depression and reproductive disorders. There is some evidence from front line Irish agencies that domestic abuse is a problem in traveller communities. It is unclear whether this is so or whether the lack of privacy afforded by a caravan means it is more public.

Mental illness

People from minority ethnic groups in Britain and elsewhere

experience high levels of mental illness, but Irish people living in Britain are more than twice as likely to be admitted to hospital with all classifications of mental illness than the indigenous population and, in most diagnostic categories, even more likely than other minority groups (Cochrane and Bal, 1987). Rates of admission for depression are higher for women than men but both exceed rates for the host population and other ethnic groups. The incidence of schizophrenia is also high, as are anxiety states and to a lesser extent personality disorders (Raleigh and Balarajan, 1992). An accurate analysis cannot be attempted without reference to patterns of mental illness in Ireland itself where the incidence of mental illness was in the 1960s considered to be among the highest in the world (Walsh and Walsh, 1968). This high rate according to Williams (1992) is not pathological but due to the greater tendency of mental illness to get beyond the resources of families and communities devastated by emigration and compromised by living in rural areas. The high incidence also relates to the availability of beds and the tendency to retain people in hospital for longer in-patient periods rather than to inherent madness.

Theories of mental illness

There is no evidence to support a genetic predisposition; selection explanations suggest a dual mechanism where a large group are positively selected for their stability leaving another group who migrate to escape. This latter group are ill-equipped to cope with the stress of migration and become ill (Cochrane and Stopes-Roe, 1979; Williams, 1992). A further explanation based on some pathogenic aspect of Irish culture has not been borne out by studies in Ireland (Walsh and Walsh, 1968; Scheper-Hughes, 1979) It is argued that mental illness in Irish people is a result of the process of colonialism and long-standing domination of Ireland by Britain (Greenslade, 1992). Drawing from the work of the Martinique born psychiatrist and political activist Franz Fanon, Greenslade proposes that the immigrant has to cope with racism, discrimination and stereotyping at the hands of the dominant culture. The central theme of Fanon's work is that members of indigenous populations of colonised countries are made to feel inferior when they reject the culture of the coloniser in favour of their own traditions. When individuals migrate they are faced with two choices.

The first is to become more like the coloniser and the second is to find a way to disappear within the host culture. Both these choices are difficult to achieve and whichever path is chosen the migrant is confronted by his/her own inferiority which induces a sense of worthlessness and despair (Fanon, 1967). Fanon's work is particularly relevant to Irish people who by their skin colour and language can remain relatively invisible. A further explanation of the incidence of mental ill health among the Irish in Britain relates to their socio-economic position and is evident in Harrison's work on alcohol, Burns and O'Meachair's work on homelessness and varius reports from Irish agencies (1988). Studies need to be undertaken, but many believe that Irish people, especially men, have difficulty expressing emotions. Examples such as bereavement and job loss are frequently cited. Although few would deny the distress of such disasters care must be taken not to neglect the everyday stresses that Irish people experience persistently and insidiously. Others would argue that repressive religious attitudes result in guilt and worth,lessness. While this may be true for some, it must be recognised that for many prayer is a comforting and healing process.

Suicide

Mortality from suicide is some twenty to thirty per cent higher in Irish people at all points in the life-span but particularly in the 20–49 age bracket (Raleigh and Balarajan, 1992). These patterns were noted some twenty years ago in Birmingham (Burke, 1976) and a relationship between suicide, socio-economic status and immigration was suggested. The picture today mirrors a worrying trend in other countries and in particular in Ireland where young people, especially men, take their lives without any hint of distress (Smith, 1995). Current research is attempting to explain this phenomenon; factors like unemployment, family breakdown, sexual abuse and changing social values are all being considered. A recent study in Ireland found a strong link between suicidal behaviour and unemployment and drug and alcohol abuse. A large number of those who attempted or successfully committed suicide had previously consulted a doctor with a mental health problem (Kelleher, 1996). However, further work must be done to examine socially conditioned psychological factors in a society where feelings and emotions are not expressed, much less discussed.

Pressure to achieve, domestic disharmony, interpersonal relationships and sexual identity may all be contributory factors. When there are no channels for emotional release young people experience great distress and see no way out. This is particularly significant for those who have left home either to get away or to advance themselves through education or employment. If they have not achieved the success expected of them or are not coping with the effort required to meet personal and family expectations they will invariably blame themselves. A feeling of not coping or of failure to achieve when compounded by a lack of social support and an absence of confidential and sensitive help all play a part in the development of mental illness.

Health of the Nation strategies for mental health note high levels of suicide in Asian women and their proposals refer to issues such as underlying cultural influences, clarity of communication, stigma and language. The Irish remain unmentioned but all the principles and even those related to language apply. Research suggests that mental health problems are fewer in areas where the Irish live in ethnic density and are able to be themselves (Cochrane and Stopes-Roe, 1979). It is also important to recognise that maintaining links with one's culture is not pathological but therapeutic (Scheper-Hughes, 1979). Culturally sensitive provision is promoted as the ideal for all minority groups, but there is a distinct resistance to Irish sensitivity and a wide- spread belief that the Irish share the same cultural values as the indigenous population. While it is recognised that older people who have been in Britain for years share many of the experiences of older English people and some older members of minority groups, many would choose specific services if a choice was available.

Awareness raising

There is a need to raise awareness of Irish issues in those who commission or provide health care. It is not sufficient to state that a large proportion of the NHS workforce is Irish, since health professionals are socialised to a western model of healthcare which neglects the values and beliefs of the client. In addition they learn to undervalue their own culture and may even be unwilling to identify with common negative stereotypes (Tilki *et al*, 1994). Irish staff, if adequately empowered, can provide culturally sensitive care, but have a particular role to play in raising awareness and enabling their colleagues to understand the cultural conventions of Irish people. They have a key role in enabling Irish people to redress some of the neglect engendered by passive acceptance of inadequate or ineffective services. The application of Fanon's work would appear to have resonance here. Apart from his analysis of the nature of oppression, Fanon suggests that feelings, of inferiority and despair can only be overcome by active participation against oppression (Fanon, 1990). In mental health terms this would mean affirming belief in one's own experience and working collaboratively with professionals towards new understandings and new responses to distress (Hopton, 1995).

Given the low self-esteem and self-effacing nature of many disadvantaged Irish people, Irish professionals and others have a responsibility to empower them to articulate their needs and demand their rights. This can only be achieved in a therapeutic partnership where client power is equal or greater than that of the professional. Irish people should take every opportunity to ensure that they are represented on the boards of commissioning agencies in roles such as that of non-executive director of NHS Trusts.

Citizen rights

Health and welfare professionals also have a responsibility to put pressure on purchasers and providers to address the needs of an 'invisible' minority who have contributed to the fabric of British society for many years and have rights as citizens of Britain and Europe. Since April 1995 health providers have been required to maintain figures for minority ethnic in-patient admissions, but few attempt to enumerate Irish people. The absence of accurate statistical data is a problem for policy makers and is difficult to rectify without a specific 'Irish' category in the census or other surveys. It is encouraging to note that as a result of persistent lobbying by the Federation of Irish Societies, the Irish are to be represented on an advisory body fine-tuning the 2001 census. It is hoped that this move will not be mere lip-service, since to date there has been little support from organisations like the NHS Ethnic Health Unit who are concerned about the needs of minorities. The recent report from the Commision for Racial Equality (Hickman and Walters, 1997) is welcome and it is hoped that the recommendations will be fully implemented. Representatives of the Irish in Britain recognise the disadvantage and poor health experienced by other minorities and support their rights to have these inequities redressed but wish to put the position of the largest and oldest group firmly on the agenda. Until official discourses recognise the 'invisible' Irish, the citizen rights to which they are entitled will continue to be eroded and their contribution to the society in which they live will not be in balance with what they receive.

References

Adelstein A, Marmot M, Dean G *et al* (1986a) Comparison of mortality of Irish immigrants in England and Wales with that of Irish and British nationals. *Irish Med J* **79**(7): 185–9

Balarajan R, Bulusu L (1990) Mortality in immigrants in England and Wales 1979-1983. In: Britton M *Mortality and Geography : a review in the mid 1980's*. OPCS Series DS No.9, London

Brody H (1973) *Inniskillane Change and Decline in the West of Ireland*. Jill Norman & Hobhouse, London

Burke A (1976) Attempted suicide among the Irish-born population in Birmingham. *Br J Psych* **128**: 534–7

Cara (1994) *Monitoring of Irish Applicants for Housing : A Survey of London Boroughs*. Cara Irish Housing Association, London

Cara (1995) *Limited Opportunities: Economic Disadvantag and Access to Housing for Single Irish Women*. Cara Irish Housing Association, London

Cochrane R, Bal S (1987) Mental hospital admission rates of immigrants to England : a comparison of 1971 and 1981. *Soc Psychiatry Psychiatr Epidemiology* **24**: 2–11

Cochrane R, Stopes-Roe M (1979) Psychological disturbance in Ireland, In England, and in Irish emigrants to England: a comparative study. *Econom Soc Rev* **10**(4): 301–20

Connor T (1987) *The London Irish: London Strategic Policy Unit*. Greater London Council, London

Crotty R (1986) *Ireland in Crisis: A study in capitalist colonial underdevelopment*. Brandon, Dublin.

Crout E (1987) Trailer bound. *Nurs Times* **83**: 12–14

Durward L (ed.) (1990) *Traveller Mothers and Babies: Who cares for their health?* Maternity Alliance, London

Fanon F (1967) *Black Skin, White Masks.* Pluto classic, London

Furnham A, Bockner S (1986) *Culture Shock: Psychological Reactions to Unfamiliar Environments.* Routledge, London

Gillam SJ, Jarman B, White P *et al* (1989) Ethnic differences in consultation rates in urban general practice. *Br J Med* **299**: 9537

Greenslade L (1992) White skins, white masks : Mental illness and the Irish in Britain. In: O'Sullivan P *Patterns of Migration.* Leicester University Press, Leicester

Greenslade L, Pearson M, Madden M (1991) Irish migrants in Britain. Socio-economic and demographic conditions. *Occasional papers in Irish studies No 3.* University of Liverpool

Harding S, Balarajan R (1996) Patterns of mortality in second generation Irish living in England and Wales: Londtudinal Study. *Br Med J* vol 312, June 1st 1996, pp1389–92

Harrison L, Carr-Hill R (1992) *Alcohol and Disadvantage Amongst the Irish in England.* Federation of Irish Societies, London

Hickman M, Walter B (1995) Deconstructing whiteness : Irish women in Britain. *Feminist Review* Summer 1995 pp 5–20

Hickman M, Walter B (1997) *Discrimination and the Irish Community in Britain.* Commission for Racial Equality, London

Hopton J (1995) The application of the ideas of Franz Fanon to the practice of mental health nursing. *Br J Nurs* **21**: 723–8

Hornsby-Smith M (1987) *Roman Catholics in England .* Cambridge University Press, Cambridge

Irish Post (1994) A catalogue of death in loneliness. 8.10.94, p7

Kelleher D, Hillier S (1996) *Researching Cultural Differences in Health.* Routledge, London

Kelleher M (1996) *Suicide and the Irish.* Mercier Press, Dublin

Lennon M, McAdam M, O' Brien J (1988) *Across the Water: Irish women's lives in Britain.* Virago, London

Linthwaite P (1983) *The Health of Traveller Mothers and Children.* East Anglia Save the Children, London

LIWC. (1995) *Rights for Travellers: A London Irish Women's Centre Survey of Local Authority Provision for Travellers in London.* LIWC, London

Lowry S (1991) *Housing and Health.* BMJ, London

Marmot M, Adelstein A, Bulusu L (1984) *Immigrant Mortality in England and Wales 1970–1978 Studies in Medical and*

Population Subjects No.47. HMSO, London

McCluskey D (1989) *Health, Peoples Beliefs and Practices.* Dublin Stationary Office, Dublin

Ni Bhrolcohain M (1990) The ethnicity question for the 1991 census: background and issues. *Ethnic and Racial Studies,* vol 13 Number 4 October 1990

Oberg K (1954) *Culture Shock.* Bobbs-Merrill, Indianapolis

Owen D (1995) I*rish Born people in Britain: Settlement Patterns and Socio-economic Circumstances.* National Ethnic Minority Data archive. University of Warwick

O Carroll I (1990) *Models for Movers; Irish Women's Emigration to America.* Attic Press, Dublin

O' Meachair G (1992) A race apart . *Social Work Today* **23**(3): 22–3

Pahl J, Vaile M (1986) *Health and Health Care Among Travellers.* University of Kent Health Service Research Unit, Kent

Pearson M, Madden M, Greenslade L (1991) Generations of an invisible minority: the health and well-being of the Irish in Britain. *Occasional papers in Irish Studies.* No 2. University of Liverpool

Positive Irish Action on AIDS (1995) *Irish People and HIV/AIDS: Advice, Information and Directory of Services.* PIAA, London

Raftery J, Jones D, Rosato M (1990) The mortality of first and second generation Irish immigrants in the UK. *Soc Sci Med* **31**(5): 577–84

Raleigh V, Balarajan R (1992) Suicide levels and trends among immigrants in England and Wales. *Health Trends* Vol 24 No 3 pp91–4

Rossiter A (1993) Bringing the margins into the centre: a review of aspects of Irish women's emigration. In: Smith A *Irish Women's Studies Reader.* Attic press, Dublin

Ryan L (1990) Irish emigration to Britain since World War Two. In: Kearney R, ed. *Migrations: The Irish at Home and Abroad.* Wolfhound Press, Dublin

Sadler C (1993) Out in the cold. *Nurs Times* **89**(16): 16–17

Scheper-Hughes N (1979) *Saints, Scholars and Schizophrenics: Mental Illness in Rural Ireland.* University of California Press, Berkeley

Smith M (1995) Lives washed away in a tide of despair. *Sunday Independent,* 7.05.95

Tilki M, Papadopoulos I , Alleyne J, (1994) Learning from colleagues of different cultures. *Br J Nurs* **3**(21): 1118–24

Vernon D (1994) The health of traveller-gypsies. *Br J Nurs* **3**(8) 969–72

Walsh D, Walsh B (1968) Some influences on the inter-county variation in Irish psychiatric hospital admission rates. *Br J Psy* **114**: 15–20

Williams R (1992) The Health of the Irish in Britain. In: Ahmad W ed. *The Politics of Race and Health.* Race Relations Research Unit, Bradford

Wilson G (1988) On the road. *Nurs Times* **84**(3): 26–7

6

Health care for refugees and asylum-seekers in Britain

Gina Taylor

Dahrendorf (1994) describes the refugee as being 'the greatest and saddest expression of the need for real citizenship' (p17). It has recently become a regular sight, when watching the television news reports, to see the frightened and distressed faces of people fleeing their homes.

This chapter concerns health care for refugees and asylum-seekers in Britain and later describes an interdisciplinary health education project which involved four local refugee communities.

Who are refugees?

Refugees are people who have been forced to leave their home country and cannot rely on the governments of their countries to protect them (UNHCR, 1994).

The term refugee has a precise legal definition. The UN convention relating to the status of refugees in 1951 stated that a refugee is a person who:

> *owing to a well-founded fear of being persecuted for reasons of race, religion, nationality, membership of a particular social group or political opinion, is outside the country of his nationality and is unable, or owing to such fear, is unwilling to avail himself of the protection of that country; or who, not having a nationality and being outside the country of his former habitual*

residence as a result of such events, is unable or, owing to such
fear, is unwilling to return to it.

(The Refugee Council,1991)

The United Nations is the international organisation that replaced the League of Nations following the Second World War with the aim of keeping peace in the world. However, this organisation is also concerned with working towards a more just world. In 1948 the General Assembly of the United Nations adopted and proclaimed the *Universal Declaration of Human Rights*. Recognition is given, in the preamble to this document, to the 'inherent dignity and the equal and inalienable rights of all members of the human family'. Over 100 states are parties to the 1951 Convention Relating to the Status of Refugees and/or the 1967 Protocol Relating to the Status of Refugees which remain powerful instruments concerning human rights. The scope of the 1951 Convention was originally confined to people who had become refugees as a result of the events that took place before 1st January, 1951, that is World War II and its aftermath. As a result of the continued movement of refugees a protocol was introduced in 1967 which made the convention universal. These two legal instruments enshrine the rights of asylum-seekers and refugees, preventing them being returned to countries where they fear persecution (Rutter, 1994). However, states differ in their interpretation and implementation of these instruments, for example, in 1995 in Britain the Home Office decided that some countries were 'safe'. Applications for asylum from these countries would be refused as it was felt that people from these countries would not face persecution if they were returned home.

The UN High Commission for Refugees (UNHCR) became operational in 1951 and is concerned with the protection of refugees and asylum-seekers and seeking longterm solutions to the problems refugees face. It is funded by donations from individual countries and its work is humanitarian and non-political. The European Convention on Human Rights also affords protection to refugees and asylum-seekers and has been used by some immigration lawyers in Europe, as it contains commitments preventing the return of people to countries where they would be subject to 'cruel or degrading treatment' (Rutter, 1994).

Most of the world's refugees have found asylum in less developed countries, in which case UNHCR provides assistance with food, shelter, medical aid and other services (UNHCR, 1994). It is estimated that only 5–10% of refugees are in developed countries, with fewer than 5% of the world's refugees in Europe.

Refugees have been arriving in Britain for many years, for example, from Eastern Europe in the late 19th century, and since then from many other parts of the world. It is estimated that some 20 million people are refugees in today's world and that 25 million are internally displaced; these are people who flee their neighbourhoods but remain in their own countries (Long, 1994). The number of refugees has doubled over the last decade.

Seeking asylum in Britain

An asylum-seeker is a person seeking safety and who is in the process of applying for refugee status in another country, for example, in Britain there are asylum-seekers waiting for the Home Office to decide whether they can remain.

Certain procedures must be followed by asylum-seekers on arrival in Britain. These are well described by Rutter (1994). People usually apply for asylum at the port of entry, which is usually an airport. Following an interview, essentially aimed at confirming the individual's identity, the asylum-seeker may be issued with a Standard Acknowledgment Letter. This states that the bearer has applied for asylum in Britain and permits him/her to apply for whatever benefits he/she may be entitled to.

The asylum-seeker will also be issued with a Political Asylum Questionnaire to complete and return to the immigration officers at the port of entry, usually within four weeks. This forms the basis of the application for political asylum with the asylum-seeker having to give details concerning the persecution faced at home. Asylum-seekers may supply evidence of risk of persecution, for example newspaper cuttings, to support their case. As the information provided in this questionnaire is fundamental to the claim for asylum, asylum-seekers are advised to seek specialist and legal advice when completing it.

Immigration officers at the port of entry have the right to detain asylum-seekers and also to refuse asylum. Britain has imposed visa requirements on some countries from which asylum-seekers originate and this clearly poses an obstacle for many. Further, Britain and some other European countries impose fines on airlines and other carriers that transport passengers who do not have the correct travel documents. Some applicants are refused admission to Britain on the grounds that they had passed through another country en route to Britain, in which case they may be returned to this third country. However, the Dublin Convention came in to force in September 1997. According to the convention applications for asylum should be made in the first European state entered by the asylum-seeker. The agreement of any third country to accept an asylum-seeker is also now required, prior to removing the asylum-seeker on the grounds that they have passed through a third safe country. However, because of differing criteria for determiniong refugees, not all European contries are considered to be safe (Shaw, 1997).

Assistance is available for asylum-seekers arriving at Heathrow Airport from the Refugee Arrivals Project. This project is based at Heathrow and is staffed by people who have themselves been asylum-seekers in the past. They can help to find accommodation, interpreters and lawyers.

Individuals who are already in Britain may apply for asylum direct to the Home Office, either in writing or in person. They will be invited for interview, and may be issued with a Standard Acknowledgment Letter and a Political Asylum Questionnaire to complete and return. Thjey must then await a decision. To hear if their application has been successful, they may wait up to two years.

If the application is unsuccessful, it may be possible to appeal. Exceptional leave to remain is sometimes granted. This is a discretionary status that may be offered to some asylum-seekers and is not the same as refugee status. Exceptional leave to remain may be granted to people whose fears of returning to their country may fall outside the UN Convention. This status does not entitle the holder to the same rights as does full refugee status and it has to be renewed at intervals. Asylum-seekers, people with exceptional leave to remain, and refugees may be required to register with the police if they are from non-Commonwealth countries and over the age of 16 (Rutter, 1994).

If granted refugee status, individuals are usually allowed to stay in Britain for four years, following which they can apply for permanent residence. Following a year's permanent residence they can apply for British citizenship provided other criteria are met.

Asylum-seekers, people with exceptional leave to remain and those granted full refugee status are entitled to the same health care as any other UK resident (Rutter, 1994). They are also entitled to other public services such as education, housing and social services. However, there have been recent changes to the entitlements for asylum-seekers who fail to claim asylum at the point of entry to Britain, and for those whose application for refugee status has been rejected and who are awaiting the result of an appeal. These people will no longer be entitled to benefits. There is concern that many asylum-seekers may be rendered homeless; and the highly controversial Asylum and Immigration Act (1996) further removes the duty of local authority housing departments to accommodate asylum seekers in priority need categories (RASU, 1996). A climate that is not seen to be supporting vulnerable groups of people may influence public opinion towards such groups resulting in racism and hostility. Spencer (1995) state that inequality in the rights and treatment of immigrants reflects a distinction in the public mind about who belongs and who does not belong.

It is important to reiterate that, even if asylum-seekers lose benefits, they will still be entitled to remain in the United Kingdom. They will also, along with those granted refugee status or exceptional leave to remain, be entitled to use National Health Services without charge. Those asylum-seekers who are not eligible for benefits may still be able to qualify for exemption from charges for prescriptions, dental treatment and sight tests, following completion of form AG1, which is available from Benefits Agency Offices, NHS hospital and health centres.

This brief account of the procedures to be followed in order to be allowed to live in Britain is intended to give an understanding of the necessary bureaucratic processes. The procedures explain reticence refugees may have in completing forms or responding to questioning relating to health care, as they may construe these as pertaining to the immigration procedures. It is also important to remember that refugees may have been in conflict with authorities in their own countries and so may be wary of statutory services.

There are fears among some people that it is becoming increasingly difficult for asylum-seekers either to seek or acquire refuge in Europe. European Union policies are being considered that aim to harmonise national visa policies, immigration controls and rules for granting asylum. The development of tighter definitions of refugee status are fuelling fears of 'fortress Europe': only those genuinely fleeing persecution by government or governmental organisations will be granted asylum (Born, 1995). Victims of civil war or those seeking refuge from violence that does not originate with the state will not be eligible.

Health care professionals and refugees

While each refugee community will display cultural differences, the groups may well share some similarities in terms of their experiences. For example, many refugees on arrival in the United Kingdom have no money, nowhere to go immediately and no warm clothes (Keaveney, 1990). Immigration is a stressful experience, even under the best of circumstances, and refugees tend to find the experience more difficult than other immigrants because they usually leave their home countries not by choice but to escape an intolerable situation (Lipson and Meleis, 1985). Because of this they often leave in a hurry, leaving many possessions, and some- times important documents, behind.

Baker *et al* (1994) believe that a greater understanding of the experience of immigration is essential. They describe a phenomenological study, conducted in Canada, to illuminate the lived experience of resettlement for a particular type of migrant – one who lacks access to an ethnic community of his or her own culture. Their informants, some of whom were refugees, describe feelings such as powerlessness, a sudden inability to understand people, bewilderment, being unsure about people's expectations, inability to understand customs and sudden feelings of being different. When questioned about their health, it was revealed that many were experiencing physical and/or emotional problems. Respondents expressed a strong commitment to adjust to the host society and were particularly receptive to support from others, actively seeking new friends and eager to establish social relationships with people from other cultures.

Any health care professional engaged in caring for refugees must have some awareness of the situations from which the refugees have fled in order to be able to understand their problems. Most refugees will have been in fear of persecution.

Persecution can take many forms. Many refugees will have been denied the right to a chosen way of life. Some may have been arrested and tortured. Some may be the victims of ethnic cleansing. The majority of refugees have fled from war. It is important to be aware that today over 85% of warfare's casualties are among civilians (Rutter, 1994).

Women refugees are particularly vulnerable, risking rape or abuse as well as persecution. In particular, refugee women may find themselves solely responsible for the welfare of the family if the male head of the family is absent. Changes in family structures and roles are likely to occur even if the male is present, for example, male roles may change drastically in the new society if the skills they relied in their home countries (perhaps agricultural) are not readily transferable to industrialised countries. In cases such as this men may find themselves unable to support their families (Forbes Martin, 1992).

Intergenerational problems can arise as children adjust to a new society. Refugee children, some of whom arrived as unaccompanied children, may find themselves in children's homes, with foster parents or in the care of a local authority. Many of these children are traumatised, suffering severe emotional problems. Tales have been told of schoolchildren hiding under tables whenever an aircraft flew overhead (Marchant, 1994). Refugee children's drawings often convey stories of trauma and pain.

Some refugees have come to Britain after having spent some time in refugee camps. These camps are often situated near the boarders of war-torn countries, as refugees often flee to neighbouring countries initially. Refugee camps may, therefore, be within range of attack. Further, such camps are often overcrowded and lacking in facilities.

Following arrival in what they might believe to be a safe country, refugees may be subjected to further discrimination and harassment on racial grounds. For example, Bosnian refugees in Essex were reported to have been terrorised by gangs of local youths (Rogers, 1994).

While many refugees come from countries where many of the people are involved in some form of agriculture, it is important to be aware that not all refugees in the United Kingdom come from nomadic or rural communities. Many will come from the main cities and will have lived in houses and driven cars. Loss of status is, therefore, another frequent problem, as refugee communities may contain people who were professionals in their own countries. These may include health professionals unable to practise in Britain because their qualifications are not recognised. Findlay (1994) comments on the economic desirability of some refugees and states that at present very little is done to foster their potential, arguing for investment in language training and support facilities to promote the integration of refugees with such potential. Rutter (1996) draws attention to the achievements of some celebrated refugees, such as Albert Einstein, Sigmund Freud and Hugh Masakela.

Four refugee groups

Asylum-seekers arrive in Britain from a wide variety of countries. Some information is offered here concerning four refugee communities who participated in a local health education project. While each of the four groups has a different cultural background, they all share the common background of leaving countries troubled by unrest.

Refugees from Eritrea

There are about 8000 Eritrean refugees in Britain, mostly located in London (Rutter, 1994). While Eritrean refugees have been arriving in Britain since the 1960s when the war with Ethiopia began, the numbers increased in 1989–90 when repression worsened. Eritrea is located to the north of Ethiopia in the Horn of Africa. This country became an Italian colony in the late 1800s and, while it was made a self-governing province of a federal Ethiopia in 1952, the Italian influence remains – some Eritreans can speak Italian and pasta features in the Eritrean diet. Eritrea's powers were gradually eroded by the Ethiopian government resulting in armed struggle for independence in the early 1960s (Donovan, 1994; Sabo and Kibiridge, 1989). During the 1970s Ethiopian government forces murdered thousands of people; the situation worsened in 1980 when both Ethiopia and Eritrea were affected by famine.

About half the Eritrean population speaks Tigrinya and a third Tigre. Other languages spoken are Arabic, Italian, English. Most Eritrean refugees in Britain speak Tigrinya. About 50% of Eritreans are Christians, belonging to the Ethiopian Orthodox Church, and the remainder are Sunni Muslims (Rutter, 1994). The literacy rate is low in Eritrea as only those living in urban areas have access to education (Rutter, 1994). It is important to be conscious of literacy: a local health education project aimed to produce an information leaflet for use among the Eritrean community, and during the course of the project it became apparent that some of the potential users of the leaflet could not read.

While agriculture provides the living for most Eritreans, most of the Eritrean refugees in Britain are from the commercial and professional middle classes, as the ability to flee to Britain is dependent on savings.

In 1993 independence was granted to Eritrea following victory for the Eritrean People's Liberation Front and a subsequent United Nations monitored referendum (Donovan, 1994). While peace has returned to Eritrea the poverty of the country is making it difficult for refugees to return (Rutter, 1996).

Refugees from Somalia

There are approximately 35000 Somalis living in Britain (Rutter, 1994). While there is a long history of Somali migration to Britain, 15000 refugees have arrived since the mid 1980s when civil war intensified. The largest Somali community is in Greater London.

Somalia is located in east Africa and has borders with Ethiopia and Kenya. Most of Somalia is semi-desert (Rutter, 1996). During the 19th century northern Somalia was a British colony and southern Somalia an Italian colony. The two countries united in 1960 when independence was gained. The Somali Republic was formed, ruled by a democratically elected government. However, by the late 1960s this government proved to be unpopular and a group of army officials seized power in a military coup. While Somali people consider themselves one ethnic group, strong clan divisions and affiliations exist and these have formed the basis of long-standing conflict following the start of the civil war in 1982. By the 1990s severe food shortages were experienced as a result of drought and disruption to farming caused by the war (Rutter, 1996). This situation resulted in thousands of deaths from starvation.

Somali is the first language of the majority of Somali people. Arabic is widely understood. The majority of Somalis are Sunni Muslims. Most of the work in Somalia (sheep, goats and cattle). The literacy rate in 1980 was 60% (Rutter, 1994).

Refugees from Sri Lanka

Over 22000 Sri Lankan Tamil refugees have arrived in Britain since 1983 and most live in London (Rutter, 1994). In Sri Lanka about 74% of the population are Sinhalese, and 18% are Tamil, thus forming a minority (Rutter, 1994).

In Sri Lanka there is a long history of separate Sinhalese and Tamil kingdoms. The island became a British colony in the early 1800s and the separate kingdoms were brought together under one administration. The British brought workers from India to work on the tea plantations: these people were described as 'plantation' Tamils and were seen as distinct from Ceylon Tamils. When Ceylon gained independence in 1948 the government was formed from the Sinhalese majority who rendered the majority of 'plantation' Tamils voteless and stateless. In 1972 when Ceylon became Sri Lanka, Buddhism (the religion of the Sinhalese people) was declared the religion of the state. In 1976 Tamil leaders called for a separate state for Tamil people and following years of mounting tension armed struggle resulted in the 1980s.

Most Sri Lankan Tamil refugees in Britain are Hindu, and a few Christians, and a few Muslims. Their language is Tamil and their literacy rate is around 90% (Rutter, 1994). In Sri Lanka, approximately half of the employment is in agriculture, fishing and forestry.

Kurdish refugees from Turkey

Over 12000 Turkish refugees have arrived in Britain since 1988; 95% of these are Turkish Kurds (Rutter, 1994). Turkish Kurds form the largest minority group in Turkey.

Most Kurds live in the mountainous areas of eastern Turkey, northern Iraq, north-west Iran and Armenia. While Kurdish history can be traced to thousands of years B.C., Kurdish national identity began to develop in the 19th century and attempts have been made at achieving an auto- nomous Kurdistan. However, in 1923 Kurdistan was divided between Turkey, Iran, Iraq, Syria and the former Soviet Union. The reaction of the Kurdish people was to rebel which evoked harsh responses. During the 1960s and 1970s Kurdish political parties were formed, calling for political independence for Kurdish people. There are an estimated 25 million Kurds forming what they claim to be the largest community in the world without a country (Born, 1996). Most Kurds live in south-eastern Turkey, and, while they form the largest minority group in Turkey, they are not recognised as a separate ethnic group, and at times have been denied certain rights, such as that of singing Kurdish songs (Budak, 1993). Such lack of recognition led to protest by members of the Kurdistan Workers' Party to which the Turkish government responded by arresting suspects and increasing its military presence (Born, 1996).

While many of the Kurdish refugees in the United Kingdom come from Turkey, it is important to realise that they may also come from other countries, such as Iraq, where in 1988 Iraqi Kurds were attacked with chemical weapons.

Most Kurdish people speak some Kurdish as it is central to their ethnic identity, as well as Turkish. The majority of Turkish Kurds are Sunni Muslims. In Kurdistan the literacy rate is 48% (Rutter, 1994). Most Turkish Kurds work on the land but Kurdistan is a mountainous region and most Kurds live in the mountainous parts of south-east Turkey forming agrarian communities with intensive social contacts in the form of extended families, neighbours and friends. Women are expected to stay at home and care for the family, including elder family members, while men are the breadwinners. As head of the family the male holds a lot of power and responsibility. However, when fleeing to seek asylum in another country Kurdish people often leave as small families. Thus, on arrival in countries of asylum, such as the United Kingdom, women tend to find that they have to perform roles that they would not normally have performed at home. Examples are shopping and taking children to school, tasks which would have previously been undertaken by another member of the extended family.

Refugees and health

Much of the literature relating to health professionals working with refugee communities comes from the United States of America. Kemp (1993), writing from experience in the United States, states that when analysing health care needs, two diagnoses common to refugees stand out: the risk of health deterioration due to barriers to access to health care; and the ineffective community coping due to lack of knowledge the of presence of services and how to gain access to them.

Rutter (1994), the Refugee Council in Britain, states that refugees have unequal access to health care and related social services. Reasons cited for this inequality include lack of knowledge of the workings of the British health care system and geographical mobility as a consequence of housing conditions in Greater London. Most refugees are to be found in Greater London. There is already a housing shortage in Britain, particularly in London where most refugees are housed in temporary accommodation in bed and breakfast hostels (Clinton-Davis and Fassil, 1992). Describing a project to help homeless people in bed and breakfast accommodation in London, Snell and McMillan (1993) report that up to 80% of families dealt with are refugees.

Clinton-Davis and Fassil (1992) describe how wherever refugees find themselves they continue to suffer from being uprooted and struggling to survive in new environments. Health and social problems extend beyond the emergency short-term phase. Further, health might not always be the first priority in a hierarchy of needs for refugees. In the initial stage of resettlement many problems are related to basic needs such as accommodation, education and employment.

Refugees tend to suffer an inordinate amount of loss which may be related to the past, the present or the future. As such, when they leave their homes, refugees might leave behind not only their material possessions, but also certain ways of life, leading Kemp (1993) to ask 'What value is the village elder in urban Paris, London or New York?' Thus refugees may suffer loss of status in the present, compounded by loss of loved ones, loss of independence and loss of community support, and further be confronted with an uncertain future.

Bernard-Jones (1992), in a preliminary study, found that in the London Borough of Haringey access to the primary care services by Somali and Eritrean refugee women was sometimes dependent on command of the English language. Not all women in the study were registered with general practitioners; some were awaiting processing of Home Office documents. There were also cultural mis-understandings. Ruddy (1992) reported significant mental distress and disease in Somali refugees in Cardiff, and also describes how help was not sought as sufferers of mental disorders were believed to bring shame upon the family.

Karmi (1992) points out that between 1988 and 1991 the number of refugees arriving in the United Kingdom rose by 500%, with London being the main destination for refugees. Because of the challenges posed to health and social services as a result of the particular problems refugees experience, Karmi recommends training for staff in refugee health: essential to this activity is the participation of the refugees themselves. As already stated, there may be members of refugee communities who have held professional positions in their own countries: such people would be ideally placed to participate in initiatives related to health and health care provision, for example, in the project described in this chapter, one of the refugee health workers was a doctor. Kemp (1993) argues that a long-term goal is healthcare independence, that is, the ability to get care without assistance. Participation is therefore essential in order that refugees can become familiar with the health services available in order to move towards independence, as well as to afford health care professionals the opportunity to learn about the needs of particular groups of refugees. Such sharing of experience should facilitate the development of rewarding relationships in health care for both users and providers of services.

Health problems can include malnutrition, chronic conditions which are exacerbated by lack of health care, and distress related to trauma. Hardie (1992) stated that tuberculosis remains an important cause of illness and death in the United Kingdom, and noted that, although annual notifications of tuberculosis had been declining, since 1987 this decline had ceased. This finding has also been reported by Raviglione et al (1993). Furthermore, notification rates are higher in metropolitan areas. Notification rates vary among ethnic groups in the United Kingdom; the highest tuberculosis notification rates are in areas with a high proportion of residents from the Indian subcontinent (Raviglione et al, 1993). Notification rates in England and Wales are 20–30 times higher in people of Indian subcontinent origin than in the indigenous white population and still higher in immigrants who have recently arrived. A recent increase in refugees from Africa and other places currently affected by conflict has also led to a rise in the number of notifications in some districts (Watson, 1993). Refugees are mostly found in metropolitan areas, particularly London, and are at increased risk of developing disease due to their vulnerability as a result of physical and mental trauma. This may be exacerbated by limited access to health care. Hardie (1992) further describes how a proportion of migrants are screened for tuberculosis on arrival at the port of entry by referral to the Port Health Control Unit. These people are then reported to districts of intended residence using the port form system. Districts are then able to offer further screening and identify those who would benefit from BCG vaccination or treatment. In the majority of districts it is only those migrants reported using the Port Forms who are screened. Hardie stressed that greater effort needs to be given to ensuring that all recent migrants are offered screening.

Working with refugee communities

The World Health Organisation (1992), within the framework of its *Targets for health for all*, addresses the theme of equity in terms of improving access to health services, and the themes of promotion of health and prevention of disease. These themes are addressed within a primary health care setting, via the medium of community participation, while ensuring intersectoral participation.

Downie, Fyfe and Tannahill (1990) describe a modern approach to health education that aims not only to prevent ill health but also to promote positive health. Such an approach goes beyond giving information to people to helping people clarify the beliefs they hold concerning health. The ultimate aim is empowerment. Such an approach is also participatory in that communication is two-way and involves understanding of people's perspectives. Effects of socio-political factors on health are recognised.

Using Tannahill's model for defining, planning and doing health promotion (Tannahill, 1985), information is given concerning preventive services and efforts are made in the domain of preventive health education by encouraging the uptake of this preventive service. According to Tannahill's (1990) preferred model for planning health education, priorities should be people and the places where they may be reached rather than diseases and risk factors. According to this model, effort is directed towards developing comprehensive programmes of health education in key community settings with key groups. Multidisciplinary and intersectoral collaboration is facilitated involving relevant gatekeepers from the start. This ensures that content, timing and methodology can be tailored to the needs and characteristics of the particular setting or group. While stressing the need for comprehensive initiatives in certain circumstances, (for example, raising awareness of the significance of preventable diseases), promotion of the uptake of specific preventive services, such as immunisation and screening, are also appropriate.

Research with refugee communities

Muecke (1992a) states that participatory research is necessary to help reduce the power differentials between researchers and refugees that silence the authentic voices of refugees. The fundamental rationale for studying a vulnerable population must be the expected value of the findings for the population.

Muecke (1992b) describes how the research designs are primarily inductive because the problems studied are ones about which little is known. It follows that ethnography and phenomenology feature prominently in research carried out with refugee groups. For refugees, realistic suspicion is a survival skill and so refugees may distrust a researcher, or for that matter any officials. Thus negotiation with an acknowledged refugee group leader to serve as intermediary is usually essential for gaining access to refugees as informants. For researchers in the health professions, that leader tends to be a trained interpreter or a health advocate at a health or social service site. Most research involves case studies with informants, or key informants who were selected purposively, in non-probability convenience or network sample recruitment methods. While this might limit the general nature of the findings, such approaches are essential for maintaining the trust of the individuals concerned and for approaching potential informants through a trusted member of their communitiy. Confidentiality and anonymity must be assured in order not to compromise the vulnerable situation of refugees. Attention is drawn in the literature to the vulnerability of refugees. This was confirmed in this project as the refugee health workers reported some suspicion on the part of the interviewees, who sometimes asked if the questions being posed were anything to do with immigration procedures. Questions were also raised as to why the particular groups were being targeted.

Lipson (1991) states that health promotion efforts cannot be effective unless they relate to the health beliefs and behaviour of the group under consideration. De Santis (1990) describes a survey administered by trained interviewers who are part of the ethnic community being studied and describes these community members as cultural informants or brokers. Lipson (1991) performed a study aimed at determining basic demographic and cultural characteristics of Afghan refugees in the USA. Such ethnographic data was acquired through interviewees and participant observation. Respondents were approached through others known to them and informal interviews took place with a convenience sample which was composed of Afghans, and health and social service professionals. The researchers were thus able to acquire knowledge regarding the informants' perspectives on their health and social needs.

Management of language differences that might arise when working with refugee groups can be achieved by blind backtranslation: a process which involves two bilingual, bicultural interpreters, A and B. A first translates the material into the language in which A is more competent; B then translates A's translation back into the source language in which B is more competent. The two versions are then compared and corrections made. Data collected during any study is then fed back to informants for their information and verification.

An interdisciplinary project with refugee communities

This section describes a collaborative and interdisciplinary project involving members of the Faculty of Health Studies, Middlesex University, New River Health Authority and representatives of the refugee communities. The aim of the project was to develop an acceptable and appropriate health education resource relating to BCG immunisation for use amongst the refugee communities in Enfield and Haringey.

Table 6.1: The refugee groups identified for this project

Refugee group	Estimated number in Haringey
Eritrean	2000
Kurdish	7000
Somalian	3000
Tamil	2500

(Source: New River Health Authority, 1994. Cited in Taylor, 1995)

The Public Health Directorate of New River Health Authority already had a Refugee Development Project in progress. This project aimed to recruit and train a team of refugee community health workers who would act as health advocates for their communities, form links with the health authority, draw attention to the priorities and concerns of the relevant communities, improve access to services and ensure that communities were seen as partners in assessing needs, planning services to meet those needs and in the delivery of health care. This project was rooted in the principles of community development. Members of this group had already identified care for the refugee communities as lack of familiarity with the English language, cultural problems with gaining access to services and poor information regarding the services available barriers to health.

The process

The idea of developing the information leaflet was initiated by a health development manager at New River Health Authority and Director of Research, Irena Papadopoulos, and Gina Taylor a senior lecturer at the Faculty of Health Studies, Middlesex University. The Commissioning and Development Manager, Health and Race, at New River Health Authority was approached to confirm the feasibility of such a project and also to ensure the involvement of the refugee workers from the four communities identified. It was also felt essential to invite the TB nurse advisers from provider units across Enfield and Haringey, as well as the Senior Consultant in Communicable Diseases, to join the steering group in order to benefit from their expert knowledge of tuberculosis. North Thames Regional Health Authority agreed to support and fund the project. Thus, various interests were represented on the steering group – representatives from the refugee communities, key staff at New River Health Authority, those of the funding agency (North Thames Regional Health Authority), professionals with expert knowledge of tuberculosis and educationalists at Middlesex University.

All major decisions relating to the progress of the project were made at steering group meetings, where concerns and issues were raised by those with varying interests.

Needs assessment

It was decided that the needs of the four refugee groups for information on tuberculosis and BCG immunisation would be identified by the four refugee health workers, following discussion with the steering group of the appropriate questions to ask. Individual interviews were held with samples of respondents who essentially formed convenience samples. The interviews were performed in community centres, social meeting places and people's homes.

Findings from needs assessment

Over 50% of the respondents from the four refugee communities knew that tuberculosis is a disease of the chest or lungs; however, 19% associated the disease with disability and death. Half of the respondents had no knowledge of BCG immunisation. The refugee health workers reported some reluctance on the part of their interviewees to discuss tuberculosis as a certain amount of stigma is attached to the disease.

The information gained from this needs assessment was used to produce an initial draft of the information leaflet, which subsequently went through several drafts prior to translation into appropriate languages. The leaflet was translated into the following languages:

* Tigrinya for the Eritrean community
* Turkish for the Kurdish community
* Somali for the Somali community
* Tamil for the Tamil community

The next stage was to pilot the leaflets. This was performed by the refugee health workers who took the leaflets to members of their respective communities and asked them to comment on the format, language, acceptability and readability of the leaflet and their understanding of it. This was achieved by posing questions and asking the respondents to rate their responses on the following scale:

Very Good	Good	Fair	Poor	Very Poor
1	2	3	4	5

The refugee workers felt that this approach was appropriate for use with their communities. The responses from this pilot of the leaflet were essentially favourable. However, some interesting issues arose. Many of the people interviewed expressed a lack of familiarity with information leaflets as these are rare in their own countries. They felt, however, that offering written information was a good idea. Some of the people interviewed, particularly in the Eritrean community, were unable to read, so the refugee worker read the contents of the leaflet to them. This was an important revelation and points to the need to assess literacy; it also identified the need to investigate the possibility of providing the information on audio-cassette tapes. Five members of the Kurdish community asked whether the immunisation was free, confirming previous findings that some refugees are not familiar with the National Health Service.

A readable formula was applied to the text of the English version of the leaflet. Ewles and Simnett (1985) describe a test based on R Gunning's FOG (Frequency of Gobbledegook) formula and adapted by the Plain English Campaign. When this test was applied to the English version of the leaflet, a score similar to that of the *Daily Mail* was obtained. This might not apply to the versions in other languages, as the calculations involve sentence length and the numbers of syllables in each word. The languages other than English involved in the production of these leaflets consist of vastly different alphabets and some of the translated texts appear longer than the English version.

Following the pilot, the content of the leaflets was translated back into English. This was a fortunate precaution as the word 'lung' had been translated as 'liver' in one of the leaflets. The accuracy of the information was again checked before the addition of illustrations and the printing of the leaflet.

The leaflets were launched at a local community centre where some of the refugee communities meet. The project team members from New River Health Authority arranged training sessions for representatives of the refugee communities who would be involved in the wider distribution of the leaflets. These sessions entailed offering more information on tuberculosis and BCG immunisation; information which could be used by these representatives when they were distributing the information leaflets.

Evaluation

The aim of the project was to develop an acceptable and appropriate health education resource relating to BCG immunisation for use amongst the refugee communities in Enfield and Haringey. The aim of evaluation is to assess the degree to which this was achieved. The results of the pilot stage indicated that the leaflets produced were indeed acceptable and appropriate for the refugee communities involved. The effectiveness of the leaflets in terms of promoting the uptake of BCG immunisation has not been assessed. St. Leger *et al* (1992) state that improvements in health from health promotional activities often become measurable only years after the event.

The project was collaborative and interdisciplinary in nature, utilising and sharing the experiences of a variety of key workers in the health care sector. Values that were essential to the progress of the project included the belief that progress should be guided by the needs and responses of the refugee groups as ultimate users of the information leaflet. Since the completion of this project North Thames Regional Health Authority has funded the translation of the information leaflet into the Bengali language and New River Health Authority has funded the translation into the Hindi and Urdu languages.

Forbes Martin (1992) stresses that refugee participation in developing and implementing programmes builds self-esteem and is cost effective as refugee participation can avoid many expensive mistakes. If refugees help with programme design the programmes will usually be more effective than if they were designed by persons unfamiliar with the society and customs. It leads to self-sufficiency and helps build values and sense of community.

DeSantis (1990) points out that the issues raised in her study are illustrated with specific reference to undocumented aliens, but that they are applicable to many other at-risk groups in general, such as ethnic minority groups, people with stigmatising illnesses and substance abusers. Moreover, while the project described here concerned four particular groups of refugees, the principles could be employed when working with many different types of minority group.

Acknowledgements

The contribution of the following to the project must be acknowledged:

Sharonn Bernard-Jones	Commissioning and Developmental Manager, Health and Race, New River Health Authority
Nevin Budak	Refugee health worker: Kurdish community
Liz Dimond	Public Relations, North Thames Regional Health Authority

Rosemary Gray	Health Development Manager, New River Health Authority
Ismail Hussein	Refugee health worker: Somali community
R Johandranathan	Refugee health worker: Tamil community
Irena Papadopoulos	Director of Research, Faculty of Health Studoes, Middlesex University
Hazel Sadler	TB nurse advisor
Dr Sheba Sen	Consultant in Communicable Diseases, New River Health Authority
Biri Tesfadet	Refugee health worker: Eritrean community
Sue Yates	Public health nurse

Since the completion of the project the New River Health Authority has become the Enfield and Haringey Health Agency and the North Thames Regional Health Authority has become the NHS Executive North Thames.

References

Baker C, Arseneault AM, Gallant G (1994) Resettlement without the support of an ethnocultural community. *J AdvNurs*, 20: 1064–72

Bernard-Jones S (1992) *Qualitative needs assessment study of Somali and Eritrean refugee women in Haringey*. Haringey Health Authority, London

Born M (1995) Asylum law made tougher. *The European*, 6.12.95. p4

Born M (1996) Nation of 25 million people fighting for a homeland. *The European*, 11-17 January, 1996 p3

Budak N (1993) *Health Needs of Kurdish Refugees in Haringey*. New River Health Authority, London

Clinton-Davis Lord, Fassil Y (1992) Health and social problems of refugees. *Social Science and Medicine*. 35(4): 507–13

Dahrendorf R (1994) The changing quality of citizenship. In: van Steenbergen B van ed. *The Condition of Citizenship*. Sage,

London

DeSantis L (1990) Fieldwork with undocumented aliens and other populations at risk. *Western J Nurs Res* **12**(3): 359–72

Donovan P (1994) Famine. *Education Guardian* 6.12.94. pp9–11

Downie RS, Fyfe C, Tannahill A (1990) *Health Promotion. Models and Values.* Oxford University Press, Oxford

Ewles L, Simnett I (1985) *Promoting Health. A Practical Guide to Health Care.* John Wiley& Sons, Chichester

Findlay A (1994) An economic audit of contemporary immigration. In: SpencerS (ed. *Strangers and Citizens. A positive approach to migrants and refugees.* Rivers Oram Press, London

Forbes Martin S (1992) *Refugee Women.* Zed Books, London

Hardie R (1992) Inner city tuberculosis: an increasing problem? *Critical Public Health* **3**(3): 21–8

Home Office (1996) *Asylum and Immigration Act.* HMSO, London

Karmi G (1992) Refugee health. Requires a comprehensive strategy. *Br M J* **305**: 205–6

Keaveney P (1990) Responding to refugees. *Nurs* **4**(2): 3

Kemp C (1993) Health services for refugees in countries of second asylum. *Internat Nurs Rev* **40**(1): 21–4

Lipson JG, Meleis AI (1985) Culturally appropriate care: the case of immigrants. *Topics in Clinical Nursing* **7**(3): 48–56

Lipson JG (1991) Afghan refugee health: some findings and suggestions. *Qualitative Health Research* **1**(3): 349–69

Long S (1994) Refugees. Issue Briefing Sheet F. *Model United Nations General Assembly Support Pack.* United Nations Association, London

Marchant C (1994) Risky future. *Community Care,* 24–30 November, 1994, pp16–17

Muecke M (1992a) New paradigms for refugee health problems. *Soc Sc Med* **35**(4): 515–23

Muecke M (1992b) Nursing research with refugees. A review and guide. *Western J Nur Res* **14**(6): 703–20

RASU (1996) *Update on benefit proposals for asylum seekers.* Refugee Council, London

Raviglione MC, Sudre P, Rieder HL *et al* (1993) Secular trends of tuberculosis in Western Europe. *Bulletin of the World Health Organisation* **71**(3/4): 297–306

Rogers L (1994) Bosnian refugees terrorised in Essex. *Sunday Times,* 4.9.94. p1

Ruddy B (1992) Any port in a storm. *Health Service Journal,* 26.11.92. p29

Rutter J (1994) *Refugee Children in the Classroom.* Trentham Books, Stoke-on-Trent

Rutter G (1996) *Refugees. We left because we had to.* The Refugee Council, London

Sabo LE, Kibirige JS (1989) Political violence and Eritrean health care. *Soc Sc Med* **28**(7): 677–84

St Leger AS, Schnieden H, Walsworth-Bell JP (1992) *Evaluating Health Services' Effectiveness.* Open University Press, Milton Keynes

Shaw J (1997) *Is There Light at the End of the Tunnel?* Amnesty International UK, London

Snell J, McMillan I (1993) Far from home. *Nurs Times* **89**(50): 39–41

Spencer S (1995) *Migrants, Refugees and the Boundaries of Citizenship.* IPPR and University of Wales Swansea, London

Tannahill A (1985) What is health promotion? *Health Educa J* **44**: 167–8

Tannahill A (1990) Health education and health promotion: Planning for the 1990s. *H Educ J* **49**(4): 194–8

Taylor G (1995) *The TB Leaflet Project. Evaluation Report.* Faculty of Health Studies Research Centre, Middlesex University

The Refugee Council (1991) *At Risk. Refugees and the Convention Forty Years On.* The Refugee Council, London

United Nations High Commissior for Refugees (1994) *Information Paper 1994.* UNHCR, London

Watson JM (1993) Tuberculosis in Britain today. Notifications are no longer falling. *Br M J* **306**: 221–2

World Health Organisation (1992) *Targets for health for all. The health policy for Europe. Summary of the updated edition September 1991.* WHO, Copenhagen

7

Developing transcultural skills

Irena Papadopoulos, Mary Tilki and Gina Taylor

Introduction

This chapter puts forward a model for transcultural care that is underpinned by the principles of anti-oppressive practice; the successful application of this model depends on a commitment to change by the whole organisation, not just by those who deliver hands-on care.

The oppressive use of professional power has been an area of debate and investigation. As long ago as 1972 Stockwell identified that some patients were more popular than others with nurses. Stockwell's evidence suggested that foreign patients, those in hospital for more than three months, those with three months previous experience of hospital, and also those with some kind of defect, for example disfigurement, featured in the unpopular groups.

Stockwell described how, in a hospital ward, nurses have power in relation to patients and so are able to define the patient's role within the ward setting. She also stated that it was to be expected that patients who do not conform to this role would be less popular than those who did conform.

More recently, Johnson and Webb (1995) revisited the issue of unpopular patients and found that it is still possible to identify popular and unpopular patients. Such popularity or unpopularity derives from the formation of social judgement, a concept the authors define as 'the apparent judgement of the social worth of persons by others' (p471).

During periods of participant observation it was found that the expression of evaluation of social worth was widespread on the ward being studied, whether in terms of 'good' and 'bad' patients or 'popular' and 'unpopular' patients.

Johnson and Webb were unable to confirm Stockwell's previous findings that personal variables such as diagnosis could be used to predict popularity or unpopularity. Instead they found that social evaluations were socially constructed within a setting of powerful influence. They describe how negative social evaluations of patients are conveyed through labelling, and how enduring such labels can be, even extending to occasions when patients were readmitted.

The tenacity of such labels has been identified by Rosenhan's (1973) classic study, which described an experiment during which eight sane people gained secret admission to different hospitals claiming to be hearing voices. On admission to psychiatric wards these 'patients' ceased pretending to be ill and behaved normally, yet they were never detected and having acquired a diagnosis of schizophrenia, each was eventually discharged with a diagnosis of schizophrenia in remission.This study demonstrated not only that once labelled schizophrenic the individuals were unable to shed the label, but also that the label attached to each individual was able to influence others' perceptions of his/her behaviour.

Labelling occurs when an individual's behaviour is not congruent with the behaviour normally expected in any given situation. As such there is little scope to allow for individuality or the fact that behavioural norms may vary both between societies and within societies.

Johnson and Webb (1995) describe how, in their study carried out in a hospital ward, nursing students were conscious of the power of some 'dominant' figures to promote a particular view of a patient.

Wilding (1982) considered the power of the professions in policy-making, resource allocation, power over people and their power to define needs and problems and concluded that the only satisfactory relationship between professions, clients and society must be one of partnership.

Hokanson Hawks (1991) undertook a concept analysis of power and for the purposes of her paper defined power as 'the actual or potential ability or capacity to achieve objectives through an interpersonal process in which the goals and means to achieve the goals are mutually established and worked toward'. Power can be both negative and positive. The positive aspect has been defined by Hokanson Hawks as 'power to', and the ability to be able to help people, while the negative aspect has been defined as 'power over', and is associated with forcefulness. An example of the former might be helping one to maintain their cultural identity while in hospital, while the latter might be forcing one to comply with the norms of the dominant culture.

Farmer (1993) in her article concerning the use and abuse of power in nursing states that, 'Failure to act on behalf of patients or to support colleagues in a fight for justice is a failure to care, and to exercise the power that is inherent in caring.' (p33)

Leininger (1988) views care as a powerful means to promote health and preserve health lifestyles, as well as being essential to curing therefore the remainder of this chapter aims to promote cultural awareness, knowledge and sensitivity leading to cultural competence. The exercises provided in this chapter are designed for individual reflection although some may be undertaken in pairs or groups. There are, of course, other ways through which you can acquire such skills: Barton and Brown (1992) describe a study that took place in the United States of America that aimed to evaluate a six-week period of student discovery learning when 'carefully screened mature nursing students' had a clinical placement with a distinct ethnic group, in this case migrant farm workers. Students of community health nursing were placed in migrant school health clinics and, through direct encounters with people, supplemented by guidelines from their teachers, the students developed respect for a cultural minority group but also were able to recognise gaps in the health and welfare systems for cultural minority groups and to discuss possible solutions.

Kemp (1993), also writing from the United States of America, describes a clinical placement of undergraduate community health nursing students with a primary care agency that serves refugees. The students engage in case finding, case management and community assessment for refugee populations. The data generated are often valuable in health planning, as well as affording the students the opportunity to learn about the culture and health needs of the groups of people concerned.

The transcultural skills development model

Almost all who have written about health care in a multi-ethnic society refer to the importance of cultural awareness and sensitivity for health professionals. Cultural knowledge is also cited as an important element in developing cultural understanding and ability to deliver appropriate care. Based on our experiences gained over the last two decades through working within the health service, through our personal research and from the available literature on this topic, we have constructed a model for the development of transcultural skills. We have identified four main concepts: cultural awareness, knowledge, sensitivity and competence. For each main concept, we have identified a number of elements or sub-concepts which need to be considered when attempting to develop or extend our transcultural skills. We have constructed a number of scenarios to help illustrate these skills and help you develop them. Naturally, there are overlaps between these concepts, and you may be able to use each scenario or activity for more than one purpose. You may question our rationale regarding the components of each main concept; the lists we are presenting are not exhaustive nor have they been scientifically developed and tested. We believe them to be a good start, an enabling tool; by focusing on these separate components we hope that you will be able to develop your skills step by step.

The first stage in the model is cultural awareness which begins with the self and an attempt to examine and challenge our own personal value base as we come to understand how these values are socially constructed. This will help us develop a questioning approach to the traditional social and health service values thus leading us to an exploration of the validity of differing views. This examination may help some staff from minority ethnic groups to express with confidence their own personal and cultural beliefs which may have been repressed by a western healthcare system (Tilki *et al*, 1994).

Empowerment, an important element of transcultural care, relies on being able to make links between our personal position and that of structural inequalities, and requires cultural knowledge and understanding. This knowledge is drawn from a number of sources but particularly from sociology which provides research evidence about disadvantage. Knowledge is also gleaned from contact with people from different groups who may be our colleagues or our clients.

Learning from them will undoubtedly contribute towards avoiding making ethnocentric judgements. However, sociology also informs debates around power, ideology and the way in which the state constructs images of normality. It particularly considers the power of the professions and the role of medicine in social control.

Cultural sensitivity can only be achieved by considering our clients as true partners, a crucial element in anti-oppressive practice (Dalrymple and Burke, 1995). Partnership demands that power relationships are challenged and that real choices are offered. These outcomes involve a process of facilitation, advocacy and negotiation that can only be achieved on a foundation of trust, respect and empathy.

The transcultural model offered in this chapter views the achievement of cultural competence as the achievement of anti-discriminatory and anti-oppressive practice. As discussed in many sections of this book, this requires health workers to recognise racism and other forms of oppression and to challenge it.

Figure 7.1: The transcultural skills development model

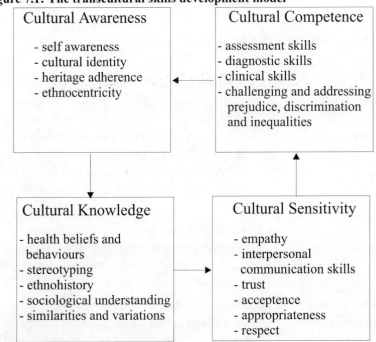

There is a growing body of knowledge which will help the reader develop the skills associated with this model. Many articles and books are given references at the end of each chapter of this book. Some specific references are made at the end of each section in this chapter.

In addition many other resources such as videos, cassettes, leaflets and teaching/study packs are available. Many of these, together with some useful addresses of organisations and government departments are listed in two very useful directories that are starred in the reference list below.

The World Health Organisation Regional Office for Europe (1992) notes that among the possible trends in a future Europe are increased migration both from outside Europe and within, and widening differences between parts of Europe and between socio-economic groups, though it is also noted that society may evolve to become more responsible and caring. It is our belief that working towards improving the health and so the life chances of disadvantaged groups of people will make for a better society for all to live in.

Developing cultural awareness

Exercise 1: developing cultural self awareness

The beliefs and practices of people from other cultures may be perceived as bizarre or irrational, yet they are no more so than some beliefs and practices of our own cultures. Some of these beliefs and practices have a direct relevance on personal health and for the ability of health care workers to provide appropriate care.

* Think of an example of a belief or a behaviour from another culture, that you might consider, or have in the past considered odd.

Comment on the exercise

You may have thought it strange that people believed in the forces of fate, spirit, curses or the power of the 'evil eye' as causes of ill health. Yet, many British people consult their horoscopes, fortune tellers, tarot readings and frequently touch wood, avoid walking under ladders or putting new shoes on the table.

Exercise 2: cultural identity/ heritage adherence

Madeleine Leininger (1991) developed an 'acculturation enabler guide' to help assess the extent of acculturation of an individual or group with respect to a particular culture or sub-culture. The enabler is an assessment tool for the traditional or non-traditional orientation of individuals. The user observes, records and rates the behaviour of an individual or groups on a five point scale, on language, cultural values, kinship, religion, politics, technology, education, environment and related areas. A short profile is then constructed which is useful for guiding decisions and actions. Below is an example, showing you how the tool is arranged. You can find the whole tool in the book *Culture Care Diversity and Universality: A Theory of Nursing* (Leininger, 1991). We recommend that you use the tool to assess yourself, a friend or a client.

Table 7.1: Rating of criteria to assess traditional and non-traditional cultural life ways or orientation

rating indicators	mainly traditional 1	moderate 2	average 3	moderate 4	mainly non-traditional 5	rater value no.
Cultural dimensions to assess traditional or non-traditional orientations 1. Language, communication and gestures (native or non-native). Notations:						
2. General environmental living context (symdols, materials and non-material signs). Specify:						

Rosenbaum (1991) used Leininger's 'acculturation enabler guide' in her study of Greek Canadian widows to assess the widows and constructed the following profile which compares first and second generation widows. (*Figure 7.2*)

Figure 7.2: Median acculturation rating and profile scale of tradition and non-traditional lifeways of first and second generation key informants (n=12)

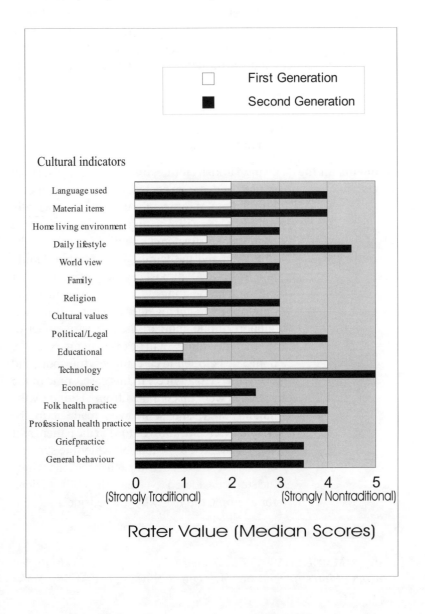

Exercise 3: ethno-centricity

A Turkish woman is in hospital for hip surgery. The surgery is performed during the morning, and by the afternoon she is lying in bed talking to her husband. She asks him if a number of family members and friends have already been to visit her. She is distressed to discover that a number of her close relatives have not yet visited her.

- Why is she concerned about her visitors?

- What may be the reason for the relatives' failure to visit?

Comments on the exercise:

In the Turkish culture, relatives and friends both expect and are expected to visit someone in hospital out of respect for the person, especially if they are very ill. Visiting is viewed as a source of moral, spiritual and practical support for the ill person and the family. For example, family and friends will almost certainly bring food for the patient; visiting a patient gives them an opportunity to get together and to reaffirm their support to one another; the closest member of the patient's family will be offered, for example, domestic help, child care, money, transport, and even 'medical advice'. In this case, some of the relatives were discouraged from visiting by the nursing staff, and some who made it to the hospital were not allowed to visit the patient as it was considered to be too soon after the surgery, or they were excluded for other reasons which the staff considered to be harmful to the patient, for example too many by the bedside.

Recommended reading

Leininger MM (ed.) (1991) *Culture care diversity and universality: A theory of nursing.* National League of Nursing Press, New York

Rosenbaum J (1991): Culture care theory and greek canadian widows. In: Leininger MM ed. *Culture care diversity and universality: A theory of nursing.* National League of Nursing Press, New York

Videos

An environment of dignity (1985). Distributed by Albany Video

Being white (1987). Distributed by Albany Video

Black and ethnic minority clients: meeting needs. Distributed by the Education Department, Royal College of Nursing (loan only)

Developing cultural knowledge

Exercise 1:   True/ False

health beliefs and   1. Hindus believe that gold worn next to the

behaviours   skin wards off disease.

2. Hindus are forbidden to practise contraception.

3. Blood transfusion and organ donation are forbidden to Hindus.

4. Roast beef and Yorkshire pudding can be eaten by Orthodox Jews.

5. All ritual laws are waived for Jewish people if life is in danger.

6. Cremation is forbidden by Jewish law

7. Muslims are allowed to take medication during the fasting period of Ramadam.

8. Menstruating women are exempt from fasting during Ramadam.

9. All Rastafarians are vegans.

10. Chewing paan is a very important custom for Bangladeshi men but not for women.

11. Chewing paan is harmless to health.

12. Post mortems are strictly forbidden within the Chinese communities.

13. Chinese people believe that the body will be weakened if too much blood is taken.

14. Older Greek people believe in the power of the 'evil eye'.

Comment on the exercise

Some people would be very critical of the above approach. Learning the answers to set questions may be called the 'recipe approach' and some would recommend that this is to be avoided as it may lead to stereotyping. We have included it here because we believe that there is a limited place for this approach. The most important thing to remember is that it is how we use the knowledge that matters. The above exercise aims to provoke thought and discussion.The answers we have provided below are generally correct though it needs to be remembered that there are individual differences as well as group variations that apply to this exercise. No matter how cultural knowledge is acquired, we all need to bear in mind that there are class, gender and age differences (amongst others), not forgetting the relevance of context. Individuals often adjust and negotiate meanings and behaviour according to the situation they find themselves in.

Answers:

1. True, 2. False, 3. False, 4. False, 5. True, 6. True, 7. True, 8. True, 9. False, 10. False, 11. False, 12. False, 13. False, 14. True.

Exercise 2: barriers to cultural sensitivity

A Greek Cypriot elderly widow is in hospital. She appears to be very quiet and sad. The nurses want to find out the reason for her sadness so that they can cheer her up. Because the woman does not speak English they find it difficult to respond to her needs through normal communication. The kind nurses decide to take an alternative approach (to be revealed shortly). Later in the afternoon, a friend of the woman visits and finds her crying. She asks her what is wrong. The elderly woman holds out her hands and shows her friend the outcome of the caring action by the nurses; they had painted her fingernails. The woman felt upset and indignant.

- Why do you think the elderly woman felt upset?

- What aspects of Greek culture were the nurses unaware of?

- What might have been the effects of the 'caring' nursing actions on the health of the woman?

Comments on the exercise

The Greek Cypriot elderly woman felt upset because she felt powerless to stop the nurses painting her nails, something that she did not want. Greek widows irrespective of age are expected to wear black clothes and no make up and to be in mourning for a long time. For elderly widows this means the rest of their lives. This is an act of respect for the dead husband. Furthermore, some of the Greek elderly women may, like women from other cultures, have never worn make up or had their hair cut or coloured. Painting one's face and nails, although widely practised by younger women, is alien to the elderly women particularly those who are widowed. Such culturally insensitive nursing actions cause distress, a feeling of invasion of dignity and loss of trust. Cultural insensitivity can have negative physiological and psychological effects. This exercise high-lights the importance of considering the sociological and anthropological dimensions of health and illness.

**Exercise 3:
stereotyping: a
barrier to cultural
sensitivity**

A middle-aged Irish man is brought into
casualty following a road traffic accident. He
smells of alcohol, is noisy and restless. He is
found dead two hours later.

* What assumptions were made about a
  man with an Irish accent and name?

**Comment on the
exercise**

The name and accent produced the stereotype of
the Irish drunk, and it was assumed his noisiness
and restlessness were alcohol induced. The
likelihood of head injury was not considered. He
was neither adequately assessed neurologically
nor observed, and died of an extradural
haematoma.

**Exercise 4:
ethno-history:
the former
Yugoslavia**

Ethno-history refers to those past facts, events,
instances and experiences of individuals,
groups, cultures and institutions that are
primarily people-centred and which describe,
explain, and interpret human lifeways within
particular cultural contexts and over short or
long periods of time (Leininger, 1991).

There are 18 million refugees in the world
today. They flee to other countries to escape
wars, ethnic conflict or human rights abuses.
Former Yugoslavia has been in turmoil for many
years and 12,000 refugees from it have arrived
in Britain since 1992.

There is no simple explanation for the conflict
that has arisen in the former Yugoslavia but the
collapse of communism in the late 1980s has
played an important part. For many centuries
Yugoslavia was divided between two great
empires, the Western and the Eastern Roman
Empires. In 1918 Yugoslavia became the
Kingdom of Serbs, Croats and Slovens. Today,
the Serbs are the largest ethnic group; the
majority of them are Eastern Orthodox
Christians. The Croats are the second biggest

ethnic group and most of them are Roman
Catholic. Bosnians are the third biggest ethnic
group and most of them are Muslims. The
various ethnic groups have been suspicious of
each other since the formation of Yugoslavia. In
1941 the Nazis invaded Yugoslavia and
thousands of Serbs, Croatian Democrats and
Jews were murdered. In 1945 Tito became
President of the country. He ruled until his death
in 1980. Tito built a relatively liberal socialist
country with an enormous army. But he failed to
solve the ethnic and regional differences, and
when he died ethnic nationalism surfaced once
again with the various regions declaring
independence. In 1991 Slovenia won its
independence but Croatia failed to as the Serb
minority resisted. Thousands of people were
killed and thousands became refugees. In 1992
the mainly Muslim government of Bosnia-
Hercegovina declared independence while the
Bosnian Serbs proclaimed their own state and
began the attack. This also resulted in thousands
of deaths and people fleeing from their homes.
All sides in the Yugoslavian conflict were
accused of carrying out 'ethnic cleansing'. By
1995 an agreement was reached about how the
former Yugoslavia will be divided and
governed.

• Think of at least six factors that may
  influence the health of a refugee from
  the former Yugoslavia. Suggest the
  reasons why knowledge of the
  ethnohistory of these refugees is
  important for health care professionals.

Comments on the
exercise

Refugees from the former Yugoslavia will most
probably be experiencing a culture shock. This
is of two types: shock and sadness at being
forced to leave their own country, and the shock
faced by anyone entering a new culture in a

foreign land. The refugees may also be going through bereavement for the loss of members of family either recently killed or left behind alive. They may even feel guilty for surviving and for escaping the fighting. Mental and physical traumas are also common. Some refugees describe that they have flashbacks and nightmares. Others may have physical war wounds such as loss of limbs and bullet wounds. Uncertainty about their status in this country will almost certainly cause stress. Living in hostels, as many of them do when they first arrive, or in other poor housing combined with no income apart from welfare benefits, add to the stress, the frustrations and the indignities they have to suffer as they find themselves having to depend on others. Language difficulties and unfamiliarity with the health and welfare system may prevent them from making use of these systems; due to this health problems may escalate rather than be prevented. Some refugees fall victim to institutional and individual racism, the existence of which is well documented.

Exercise 5: ethno-history: the holocaust

An elderly Jewish woman was admitted to a ward for the care of elderly people as she was becoming increasingly disorientated. The woman became very distressed when carers attempted to take her to the bathroom. The woman's son revealed that during the Second World War his mother had been held in a concentration camp and he suggested that some of her distress might stem from memories of this experience.

- Consider some of the events this woman may have witnessed or experienced which may have added to her distress.

Comments on the exercise

Throughout history Jewish people have been persecuted and discriminated against. Anti-semitism still exists around the world today and Jewish people have been used as scapegoats for troubled nations. While such sentiments existed prior to the Second World War, it was during this period that Hitler as a powerful leader was able to inflame hatred of Jewish people, enacting laws against them and depriving them off jobs and property. On the 9th–10th November 1938, Nazis throughout Germany attacked Jewish shops and synagogues. This night was known as 'Kristallnacht' the night of the broken glass. Following this, thousands of Jewish men and boys were rounded up and taken to concentration camps. Such events prompted many Jewish families to flee Germany, though some other countries restricted the numbers of Jewish refugees they would accept. In spite of the fact that many Jews in Germany were cultured, assimilated and active contributors to the national life of Germany (Gilbert, 1987), for those who remained life became increasingly difficult as their rights became progressively eroded. As war progressed and German occupation of other European countries spread, steps were taken to make Jewish people easily identifiable, for example, requiring them to wear a yellow Star of David. Acts of terror, hostility and discrimination, as well as deprivation of citizenship, were no longer confined to Germany. Concentration camps were built in Germany initially and then in neighbouring occupied countries to house opponents of Hitler and people who were considered inferior. Extermination camps were built as part of a systematic campaign to exterminate Jewish people. Jewish people were transported by train to these camps. The trains were crowded and prisoners were given nothing to eat or drink. Many were not told where they were going. On arrival at the camps there was often selection: some prisoners were selected for labour, others for gassing. Those destined to be killed were led to huts where they were asked to undress before going to bathrooms which would be subsequently filled with gas. The bodies were burned. Some whose lives were initially spared were used for inhumane experiments. Many died of starvation and illness. By the end of the war, about six million Jews had been murdered. While these events happened a long time ago, there are of survivors of the concentration camps still alive.

Accounts of atrocities and ethnic cleansing in former the Yugoslavia have displayed similarities to the concentration camp experiences of the Second World War.

Exercise 6: sociological understanding

Care that is acceptable to members of specific groups requires understanding of and respect for lifestyle, community, and sociocultural orientations as the context for health promotion, maintenance, and restoration (Kavanah and Kennedy, 1992). Sociology is the study of human societies that imply historical, anthropological and critical sensitivities (Giddens, 1986).

- Think of an example that illustrates the usefulness of 'sociological understanding'to the health care professional.

Comments on the exercise

You may have thought about issues of the family. For example, how you and others define it, what are the most important relationships within the family, by whom or how are decisions normally made, the role of the women in different families, and how children are viewed and cared for?

Knowing about these issues is important for all health care professionals, as they all affect health and health behaviour. And while complete knowledge is not possible (indeed it may not even be the goal), general knowledge about these issues provides a useful framework for action.

Exercise 7: similarities and variations

Helman (1990) describes a set of commonly held beliefs about colds, chills and fevers in a London suburb. These beliefs are widespread throughout Britain and are shared by many ethnic groups. Rain or damp environments cause colds like a 'cold in the head' or a 'runny nose'. Cold but dry conditions cause a feeling of cold such as aches and pains and shivering. Chills occur either below the waist (a chill in the kidneys) or above it (the stomach, the head chest and sinuses). These conditions are believed to be caused by careless behaviour such as going out after a bath or sitting in a draught. Victims get little sympathy and are expected to care for themselves by restoring warmth, staying in bed, having hot drinks and warm food. By contrast, fevers are believed to be caused by invisible agents which penetrate the body. These agents exist in the air and travel between individuals; they give rise to many symptoms in those who fall victim to them. The sufferers are blameless and are encouraged to drink plenty to 'flush' the germs out, to starve them or exterminate them by antibiotic treatment.

• How would you reassure the parents who worried that their pyrexial child would 'catch a chill' if h/she was fanned?

Comments on the exercise

This is an example of a set of beliefs shared amongst a number of cultural groups and the indigenous population. Despite the focus of this book on the different cultural health beliefs and health practices of minority ethnic groups, we must remember that there are more similarities between groups than there are differences. However, we must also remember that the small differences that exist are very important. Perhaps you can consider the following: problems may occur when a child with a fever is kept warm in the belief that it is the best way to treat it. Occasionally despite the best efforts of health practitioners some parents see sponging, light clothing or fanning as dangerous and will keep the child wrapped up.

Recommended Reading:

Commission for Racial Equality and Age Concern (1995) *Age and Race: Double Discrimination. Life in Britain Today for Ethnic Minority Elders. Health.* CRE, London

Giddens A (1986) *Sociology. A brief but critical introduction.* 2nd Ed. Macmillan, Basingstoke

Gilbert M (1987) *The Holocaust. The Jewish Tragedy.* Fontana, London

Helman CG (1990) *Culture, Health and Illness.* Butterworth Heineman, Oxford

Kavanagh K, Kennedy PH (1992) *Promoting Cultural Diversity. Strategies for Health Care Professionals.* Sage, Newbury Park

Jayaratnam R (1993) The need for cultural awareness. In: Hopkins A, Bahl V *Access to Health Care for People from Black and Ethnic Minorities.* Royal College of Physicians, London

Karmi G (ed.) (1992) *The ethnic health factfile. A guide for health professionals who care for people from ethnic backgrounds.* North West/North East Thames RHA, London

Karpf A (1966) *The War After: Living with the Holocaust.* Heinemann, London

Rutter J (1996) *Refugees. We left because we had to* 2nd ed. The Refugee Council, London

Van der Rol R, Verhoeven R (1993) *Anne Frank. Beyond the Diary.* Viking, London

Wouk H (1978) *War and Remembrance.* Fontana/ Collins, Glasgow

Videos

Meeting Hindu families (1992). Distributed by Southern Derbyshire NHS Trust

Meeting Muslim families (1992). Distributed by Southern Derbyshire NHS Trust.*Meeting Sikh families* (1992). Distributed by Southern Derbyshire NHS Trust

Why you need to know about thalassaemia (1990). Distributed by UK Thalassaemia Society

The social care needs of Afro-Caribbean elders. (Haringey Council). Distributed by N. Films

Films

Schindler's List

The Diary of Anne Franks

Visit

The Jewish Museum, Raymond Burton House, 129–131 Albert Street, Camden Town, London NW1 7NB, Telephone 0171 284 1997

Developing cultural sensitivity

Exercise 1: empathy

Kalisch (1971) defined empathy as the ability to perceive accurately the feelings of another person and the ability to communicate this understanding to him or her. Tschudin (1989) stated that empathy is not something magic, which you either have or have not. Empathy can be learnt; empathy is the basis for any kind of helping.

• Do you agree with Kalisch's definition and with Tschudin's affirmation? If you do, make a list of prerequisite skills or factors which, in your view, are necessary to develop empathy. If you do not agree, how would you enhance either the definition or the affirmation?

Comments on the exercise

Your list might include some of the skills identified by Tschudin such as: respecting, staying open, attending, using open questions, giving permission, being non-judgmental. Based on the arguments presented in this book and our model, we would add the following: cultural awareness, cultural knowledge and cultural sensitivity. We believe that these important elements will enhance the concepts of empathy encompassed by the above statement.

Exercise 2: empathy and trust

In a recent study into the health needs of the Greeks and Greek Cypriots living in London, Papadopoulos (1996) found that the majority of the participants preferred to be cared for by a health professional who shared their ethnic background. This response was given by individuals of all generations who explained that their preference was base on a mutual under- standing of the Greek culture which made them feel more comfortable with the care giver. Being able to identify with the carer enables the client to feel more secure in the knowledge that the carer has a deeper understanding, one which goes beyond the spoken words. This phenomenon was reported by other cultural groups. Farooqi (1993) reported that many Asian patients choose Asian physicians.

Eleftheriadou (1994) describes the case of Stella, a Greek client in her mid-twenties, who sought counselling because she was experiencing problems in adjusting to the British culture. Although she always spoke to her in English (even though she knew that the counsellor spoke Greek), she told the counsellor that she would not have come to counselling had she not had a counsellor from the same culture.

She told the counsellor that because of the commonality of culture, she was more to her than a counsellor but also a friend and a fellow Greek who understood 'the behaviour of us Greeks'.

* Bearing in mind the preferences of clients on the one hand and the current and future provision of health care on the other, what do you see as problems and how can these be overcome?

Comments on the exercise

The are two main issues associated with the above. Firstly, it is unlikely that we will ever reach a situation when all clients will have the carers of their choice. We may even ask whether this is the desired model to follow; we are sure you can think of reasons why this should or should not be the desired model. (See Smaje's book on *Health Race and Ethnicity* for an informed discussion on this topic.) Secondly, the reality is (and will remain for the foreseeable future) that recruitment patterns are unlikely to change dramatically, thus the majority of carers will be from the indigenous population. It is therefore important to improve the cultural competence of all carers while at the same time encouraging a better representation of certain ethnic communities within the caring professions.

Exercise 3: interpersonal/ communication skills

Racism or 'ethnicism' is reproduced through everyday talk and interpersonal enactment in everyday communicative situations (van Dijk, 1987). We asked a group of students to tell us some examples of commonly held stereotypes that they had observed in others and that had acted as barriers to forming good relationships with clients from minority ethnic groups or had interfered with the communication processes (Papadopoulos *et al*, 1995). These are some examples:

If a person cannot speak good English s/he is often treated as though s/he is not very bright.

Irish people are thick.

Most black people have lots of children and are depend on the State.

Black people make too much fuss about too little pain.

Indian parents do not want to stay with their sick children in hospital as they have shops to run.

Most Nigerians are infected with the HIV virus.

* How would you tackle these stereotypes in a way that promotes effective interpersonal relationships and communication?

Comments on the exercise

Our students suggested the following strategies: Confront those who make jokes about the way you speak or about your accent. Do not justify racism or discriminatory behaviour by saying that it goes on all the time. Encourage individuals to get to know persons from other cultures. Acknowledge that people fear the unknown but that this does not excuse their exhibiting harmful behaviour towards others. Try to focus on facts. Act in ways which promote good communication.

Exercise 4: interpersonal communication skills

Complete the following statements:

a. Eye contact is a sign of..

b. Shaking hands is a sign of..

c. Kissing and embracing is a sign of..

d. Talking about you achievements is a sign of..

Comments on the exercise

a. The meaning of eye contact varies from one culture to another. In Western cultures it is a sign of listening, associated with honesty and genuineness. In some Asian and African cultures direct eye contact is considered rude in certain circumstances such as when the status of the two individuals is different or when a woman greets a man.

b. Greetings vary from one culture to another. (Eskimos rub noses when they meet.) Rituals around handshaking vary considerably. In Britain shaking hands is a formal way to greet someone one has just met, while in France and many other Mediterranean countries people shake hands with those they have met several times even on the same day.

c. In northern European and many Asian countries kissing and embracing tend to be reserved for close friends or relatives. Men would not normally kiss their male friends or relatives when they meet. In Middle Eastern cultures, it is common for men to kiss and hug each other as a form of greeting.

d. British and Irish people are not encouraged to be boastful about their achievements whereas European Americans, for example, consider talking about their achievements as a very positive act and are therefore less reticent in talking about themselves.

Exercise 5: acceptance

Skills related to acceptance are of two kinds: those that help us develop self-acceptance and those that help us accept others. Knowing and accepting ourselves enables us to accept others, a necessary component of interpersonal communication and relationships. Below there is a list of selected articles from the *Universal Declaration of Human Rights* (1948).

• Read each article and consider your true personal views and attitudes about it. Think of practical examples in which each article applies to you and to others. Have you ever had any experiences in which you lost your human rights? How did these make you feel? Can you recall instances from your professional life in which others lost their human rights? How did these make you feel? If possible discuss this exercise with a friend. Receiving feedback about our attitudes and feelings is a good way of improving ourselves.

Article 1: All people are born free and equal and should behave with respect to each other.

Article 2: Everyone should have the same rights regardless of their race, colour, sex, nationality, religion, political opinion or social origin.

Article 3: Everyone has the right to live in freedom and safety.

Article 7: Laws must not treat people differently because of their race, sex or way of life.

Article 13: Everyone has the right to travel and live anywhere in their home country. A person also has the right to leave any country, including his or her own, and to return to it.

Article 14: People have the right to ask for asylum in another country, if they fear persecution. A person loses the right to ask for asylum if he or she has committed a serious non-political crime, and has not respected the Universal Declaration of Human Rights.

Article 15: Everyone has the right to a nationality.

Article 17: Everyone has the right to own property. No-one can take other people's possessions without a fair reason.

Article 18: Everyone has the right to think and believe in what they want, this includes the right to practice a religion.

Article 19: Everyone has the right to express their thoughts, whether by speaking or in writing.

Article 22: Everyone has the right to social security. This includes shelter, health care and enough money with which to live.

Article 25: Everyone has the right to a decent standard of living. Those who cannot work should receive special help. All children, whether born outside marriage or not, have the same rights.

Exercise 6: appropriateness

A young orthodox Jewish woman has had her fifth child in seven years and the doctor proceeds to advise her about contraception. The woman is uncomfortable and embarrassed and although she does not want another child she reuses the offer of contraception.

• How might the doctor's intervention have been culturally inappropriate?

Comments on the exercise

Family planning is considered a private matter between the couple and if required would be discussed by both partners with the practitioner concerned. In addition a large family is seen as a blessing and motherhood and child rearing are highly valued activities.

Exercise 7: respect

A client from Mauritius is admitted to the unit where you are the person in charge. As you introduce her to other staff some say 'I will never be able to pronounce that' or 'I'll never remember such a strange name'. One member of staff suggests using a nickname or a shorter version of her name. You observe that the client is not impressed but does not say anything.

• How will you address the issue of clients' names at the next staff meeting?

Comments on the exercise

Name is an important part of identity and we all have a preference as to whether we use our full name, a short version of our name or a different name altogether. We feel slighted when somebody forgets our name, gets it wrong or uses a form which we don't like. We dislike it when people are either too familiar or too formal. This client may have similar feelings about her name. If a name is difficult to remember or pronounce, it would help to get the person to repeat it. It also helps to write it down phonetically and you may wish to make a note of that in the client's records. In addition older people often prefer to be addressed more formally. British people may prefer to be addressed as 'Mr' or 'Mrs'. In other cultures there are other conventions to show respect. For example, older Turkish people would be addressed by their first name followed by 'Hanim' for a woman and 'Bey' for a man as in

Fatma Hanim or Ali Bey. Greek people generally use their first name with the 'Mr' or 'Mrs' prefix. For example Mrs Eleni or Mr Andreas. To be more precise, the term 'Kirios' is used instead of 'Mr' as in 'Kirios Andreas' whilst the term 'Kiria' is used instead of 'Mrs' as in 'Kiria Eleni'.

* Ask friends or colleagues who are from different ethnic backgrounds from your own how they use names and terms of address.

Recommended reading

Eleftheriadou Z (1994) *Transcultural Counselling.* Central Book Publishing, London

Farooqi A (1993): How can family practice improve access to health care for black and ethnic minority patients? In: Hopkins A, Bahl V ed. *Access to Health Care for People from Black and Ethnic Minorities.* Royal College of Physicians, London

Kalish BJ (1971): Strategies for developing nurse empathy. *Nursing Outlook* **20**(3)

Papadopoulos *et al* (1995) *Teaching Transcultural Care. An investigation into the teaching methods suitable for transcultural education for nurses and midwives.* Middlesex University, London

Papadopoulos I (1996) *Health Needs of the Greek and Greek Cypriots Living in London.* Unpublished PhD thesis

Tschudin V (1989) *Beginning with Empathy. A learners' Handbook.* Churchill Livingstone, Edinburgh

van Dijk T (1987) *Communicating Racism. Ethnic Prejudice in Thought and Talk.* Sage, Newbury Park

Videos

The right to be understood: a training video on working with community interpreters (1987). Distributed by Concord Video and Film Council

Facing the challenge (1992). Distributed by Ceddo Film/Video

Death with dignity: meeting the spiritual needs of patients in a multicultural society. Distributed by Macmillan Magazines

Blood disorder not disease (1989). Distributed by Verite a Tous

Black and ethnic minority clients: meeting needs (1993). Distributed by Healthcare Productions

Developing cultural competence

Exercise 1: assessment skills

The breast care specialist practitioner is called to see an Indian woman who needed persuasion to be fitted for a prosthesis following mastectomy. She is now reluctant to wear the prosthesis. The patient's care plan suggests that she shows little interest in her appearance and may well be depressed.

• What questions might the specialist practitioner ask and why?

Comments on the exercise

The specialist practitioner would discuss the patient's feelings first but would ask questions about the patient's preference for western or traditional Indian dress. Women who wear the sari frequently do not wear a bra preferring a short bodice. The folds and drapes of the sari which goes over the bodice hides the contour of the breasts. Since the majority of breast prostheses require a bra, this would create an additional problem for the Indian woman who normally wears the sari.

Exercise 2: diagnostic skills

One morning, at breakfast time, an eighteen month old boy reached just that little bit farther than he had ever reached before and got hold of a cup of tea which fell over and spilled over his body causing extensive scalding. His distressed parents rushed the little boy, who was blond and fair skinned, to his local accident and emergency department where he received initial emergency treatment and was then transferred to the regional burns centre.

Meanwhile, on the other side of town, another little boy met with a very similar accident. When his distressed parents took him to the local accident and emergency department he was sent home, following initial treatment. This little boy was of Asian origin and the severity of the scalds was underestimated. He was eventually transferred to the regional burns centre, after being taken to the accident and emergency department for the second time by his parents who were worried about his deteriorating condition. However, valuable time had been lost. Both little boys made a good recovery and were eventually discharged home.

- Any inflammation will be more easily observable on a fair skin than on a darker skin. Consider the skills that can be employed and developed in order to assist in the assessment of injuries of the little Asian boy.

Comments on the exercise

Particular attention must be paid to the history of the injury, thus listening and questioning skills will be employed during the assessment of the patient. Observing and recording the vital signs is as usual of great importance as they may give indications of the severity of the injury which may not be immediately apparent on initial observation of the wound(s). In order to develop observation skills in instances such as this, it is advisable tactfully to make use of every available opportunity to make close observation of patients with such wounds. Also, while the pallor might not be immediately apparent when looking at the skin, observations can be made of mucous membranes. Do ask a colleague to confirm the diagnosis you have made about the nature and extent of the health problem. Reflecting on the way you have handled a situation, including the assessment and identification of problems, is a very positive and beneficial way to achieving cultural knowledge, skills and competence.

Exercise 3: clinical skills

A strict Muslim patient has had a stoma fashioned during elective surgery. Although he appeared quite well prepared pre-operatively he refuses to participate in caring for his stoma post-operatively. His English is poor and, despite translating through professional interpreters, he is adamant in his refusal to touch the stoma.

• Why might the patient, who appeared to understand pre-operatively, has such difficulty after surgery?

Comments on the exercise

All patients experience anxiety when first required to handle their stoma or related appliances. It is more problematic for Muslim patients who do not use the right hand for toilet purposes. Although single handed appliances are available for those who are unwilling or unable to manage their stoma with two hands, the immediate post-operative period requires the use of both hands. Nurses must be sensitive to this and recognise that it will take longer to promote independent self care. Encouraging the patient to use the left hand to hold the appliance or to assist in cleaning is advised. Care must be taken to avoid contaminating the right hand in any way so that the patient can feel confident that in time he will be able to manage the appliance.

Exercise 4: clinical skills

For many years all Western health behaviours and medical practices have been assumed to be superior to those of other cultures. People from minority ethnic communities have been encouraged to adapt to and adopt these practices.

• Identify one practice common in non-Western cultures which was avoided or frowned upon, but which has been proved to be appropriate.

Comments on the exercise

Traditionally Middle Eastern women have always laid their newborn babies on the back or side. Midwives and health visitors in the UK have been discouraging this practice in the belief that lying on the stomach was safer for the baby. It has recently been established that lying babies on their back or side is much more effective in preventing cot deaths.

Exercise 5: challenging and addressing prejudice, discrimination and inequalities

McNaught (1985) characterised racial discrimination in the following terms:

1. Patient reception and handling: Patients from minority ethnic groups were kept waiting longer than other patients. Staff were addressed patients in a derogatory or racist manner for example, 'Sunshine', 'Sam' etc.

2. Clinical consultation: Poor or no explanation of treatment or care. Assumption that these patients were 'faking' their symptoms or that they were hypochondriacs. Inappropriate or delayed treatment.

3. Patients' consent to medical treatment: Inadequate explanations. Exceeding procedures or treatments without further consent or explanation.

4. Nursing care: Offhand treatment. Racist slurs or comments. Unnecessary medication, particularly of the mentally ill. Denying patients medicine on the grounds that ethnic minorities 'have a low pain threshold'.

5. Health surveillance/diagnosis: Using para-meters and behavioural models that are culturally specific to white British people.

- The above statements were made more than ten years ago. Think of your work experiences in the last six months. Which of the above discriminatory/racist situations still exist? What are the reasons for not making much progress in the areas you have identified. In which areas have improve- ments been made and why?

- How familiar are you with the *Race Relations Act 1976*?

Comments on the exercise

It is sad to say that much discrimination and racism still exists in the NHS. Political correctness has made us all more aware about what is acceptable, particularly regarding the language we use. You may have concluded that patients are no longer addressed inappropriately. However, you will probably also conclude that much other discriminations still remains. For example, recently, some of our students described how women in labour (who could not speak English) were either not offered epidural pain control – even though they might have benefitted from it – or were given this method of pain control with very little explanation which may not have even been understood. Much indirect and hidden discrimination is tolerated by many professional carers for many and complex reasons. Ignorance, lack of training, shortages of staff and other resources are some of those most commonly cited. The personal belief held by many professional care providers that the responsibility belongs to those members of minority groups who fail to learn the English language or who continue with their cultural practices is perhaps one of the most significant factors that stops the development of positive attitudes. The *Race Relations Act 1976* states that it is unlawful to discriminate on racial grounds, either directly or indirectly. Racial grounds are race, colour, nationality, and ethnic or national origins.

- **Direct discrimination** is defined as treating a person less favourably than another on grounds of race.

- **Indirect discrimination** is when, although a condition is applied equally to all people, a considerably smaller proportion of people from racial groups can comply with it than others, and which cannot be shown to be justifiable irrespective of colour, race, nationality or ethnic or national origin of the person to whom it is applied.

- **Victimisation** occurs when a person receives less favourable treatment than others in the same circumstances because it is suspected or known that s/he has brought proceedings under the Act or given evidence or information relating to such proceedings or alleged that discrimination has occurred.

- **Racial harassment** involves physical and/or verbal abuse or other types of behaviour which deters people from using NHS services.

Recommended reading

McNaught A (1985) *Race and Health Care in the UK*. Health

Education Council, London

The Race Relations Act 1976. HMSO, London

Commission for Racial Equality (1992) *Race Relations Code of Practice in Primary Health Care Services.* CRE, London

Papadopoulos I, Worrall L (1996) *All health care is good until you have a problem: An examination of the primary health care needs of the Greek and Greek Cypriot women.* Greek and Greek Cypriot Women of Enfield, London

UN (1948) *Universal Declaration of Human Rights.* Geneva

Videos

Mistaken for mad (1990). Distributed by Healthcare Productions

Depression in ethnic minorities (1991). Distributed by CFL Videos

According to need: services for older people in a multiracial society (1989). Distributed by Age Concern England

References

Barton JA, Brown NJ (1992) Evaluation study of a transcultural discovery learning model. *Public Health Nursing.* **9**(4): 234–41

Dalrymple J, Burke B (1995) *Anti-Oppressive Practice. Social Care and the Law.* Open University, Buckingam

Farmer B (1993) The use and abuse of power in nursing. *Nursing Standard*, **7**(23): 33–6

Health Education Authority (1994) *Health Related Resources for Black and Minority Ethnic Groups.* HEA, London

Hokanson Hawks J (1991) Power: a concept analysis. *J Adv Nurs* **16**: 754–62

Johnson M, Webb C (1995) Rediscovering unpopular patients: the concept of social judgement. *J Adv Nurs* **21**: 466–75

Kemp C (1993) Health services for refugees in countries of second asylum. *International Nursing Review* **40**(1): 21–4

Leininger MM (1988) Leininger's theory of nursing: cultural care diversity and universality. *Nursing Science Quarterly* **1**(4):152–60

Rosenhan DL (1973): On being sane in insane places. *Science* **179**: pp250–9

Stockwell F (1972) *The Unpopular Patient.* RCN, London

Tilki M *et al* (1994) Learning from colleagues of different cultures. *Br J Nurs* **3**(21): 1118–24

Wilding P (1982) *Professional Power and Social Welfare.* Routledge and Kegan Paul, London

World Health Organisation Regional Office for Europe (1992) *Targets for health for all. The health policy for Europe. Summary of the updated edition.* World Health Organisation Regional Office for Europe, Copenhagen

8

Conclusion

Gina Taylor, Mary Tilki and Irena Papadopoulos

The preceding chapters have attempted to take a somewhat different stance to a subject about which a body of literature already exists. The text has taken a broad approach which embodies multiculturalism and anti-racism and is firmly located in a context of citizenship. This stance seeks to challenge explanations that blame poor health on cultural lifestyle factors and acknowledges the ways in which disadvantage is socially produced and exacerbated by citizenship status. Despite an abundance of research and scholarly work there are still groups about which very little is published. There is also a dearth of detail that relates to the experience of belonging to a minority ethnic group, and especially in relation to health and illness. The chapters on Greek and Irish people and refugees attempted to address just two of these deficits.

The chapters in this book raise more questions than answers and argue the need for further research. Much more information is needed about the experience of ill health and access to health care for minority ethnic groups. There is a need for research that provides for a greater understanding of health beliefs and behaviours and a more detailed examination of the mechanisms that underlie patterns of ethnic health. It is also crucial that appropriate assessment of need and evaluative studies are undertaken and that the findings are used in strategic planning of services for people from minority groups.

The health reforms of the 1980s and 1990s might at first sight projects a bleak picture for people from minority ethnic groups but despite their flaws, such as decentralisation and market principles, they could provide openings for the development of equal opportunities (Mason and Jewson, 1992). While the nature and purpose of Britain's welfare system have been fiercely debated during the 1980s and 1990s, there has been a convergence in the language used in this debate with citizens' charters and citizens' rights being discussed across the political spectrum (Coote, 1992). This emphasis on the concept of 'service user' will inevitably mean changes in professional practice. Pietroni (1994) discusses how the anxieties that may be generated by such changes may bring health and welfare professionals together in joint planning initiatives. Leathard (1994) views one of the challenges of interprofessional work as an opportunity to address discrimination and equal opportunities. Service contracts provide scope for standard setting and evaluation and should include an ethnic dimension relative to the local area. Services might be developed to meet the particular health needs of minority clients such as hypertensive clinics specifically catering for those from Afro-Caribbean groups. Language and advocacy services would enhance the quality of provision and increase uptake. The role of the independent and voluntary sector could be extended and secured by joint planning and provision to meet the needs of different cultural groups.

Decentralisation and self government might lead to a decline in the enforcement of equal opportunities policies through local interpretation or application. However, this freedom allows trusts and agencies opportunities for the recruitment of staff from minority and other disadvantaged groups to meet their particular needs. This may be through the employment of ancillary or professional staff with language or advocacy skills or through engaging suitable members of particular communities to work collaboratively in the provision of health promotion or other projects.

Anti-discriminatory principles can redress some of the failures of the past by recruiting and ensuring the development of staff from minority groups. Such staff, when adequately empowered, can contribute to the cultural sensitivity of the organisation. It has been argued that equal opportunities policies and affirmative action have had limited success because they were seen more as an end in themselves than as the policy development tool they were. They rarely identified what the goals were or what a diverse organisation or service could look like. Historically, the focus of change was on disadvantaged groups rather than the internal and external environment of the organisation (Behrens and Auluck, 1993). The provision of training alone for minority staff will not solve the problem entirely as it does not address the context of racism and discrimination within which they work (Behrens, 1993).

By focusing on 'managing diversity' rather than on equal opportunities (Behrens and Auluck, 1993; Kandola, 1993) the benefits for the organisation are emphasised rather than the needs of disadvantaged groups. Although the breadth of focus is different this approach shares many of the same initiatives of equal opportunity approaches (Kandola, 1993). Managing diversity seeks to maximise the potential for all staff to enhance their contribution to the organisation and has benefits for individuals and the service as a whole. It embraces all employees and potential employees, not just personnel and human resources staff, and requires a commitment from everybody. Managing diversity concentrates on the culture of the organisation and its objectives. Managers are particularly required to take the lead in equality strategies and to improve the skills of staff so they can contribute to the organisation by their own personal development. It also seeks to ensure a workforce which represents the community it serves and from which its customer base is drawn.

On several occasions in this book the term 'empowerment' has been mentioned. This is a complex issue; concept of 'empowerment' is fraught with problems at both a theoretical and practical level.

Gibson (1991) defines empowerment as follows:

In a broad sense, empowerment is a process of helping people to assert control over the factors which affect their lives. This process encompasses both the individual responsibility in health care and the broader institutional, organisational or societal responsibilities in enabling people to assume responsibility for their own health. (p354)

In her concept analysis of empowerment Gibson identifies that the term has psychosocial, political and ethical connotations and that it may be easier to understand in terms of its absence, for example, in terms of powerlessness or oppression. Drawing on the work of several authors, Gibson states that empowerment is a positive concept, addressing people's strengths, rights and abilities, rather than deficits and needs. It is also dynamic, involving a giving of power by one party and the taking of power by another. Thus, Barnes and Walker (1996) state that authority deriving from professional knowledge is balanced by authority deriving from the experiential knowledge of the user, thus rendering empowerment a collaborative process. As power is located in the expertise of health care professionals, self understanding is a pre-requisite for empowering others. Health professionals therefore need skills in teaching and counselling and in coordinating multi-disciplinary teams in order to facilitate the empowerment of others. It is also important to be able to address the conditions in society that mediate health or ill health, as well as giving consideration to the individual service user. Braye and Preston-Shoot (1995) therefore advocate the use of holistic models for empowering practice, which aim to gain a personal understanding of how any individual's experience is constructed by his/her position in society. Such models would seem to reinforce the need to draw on the experiences of health care professionals from differing backgrounds in order to share perspectives that result from being located in a variety of positions in society.

There is a powerful legacy of professional socialisation that may foster barriers to empowerment which may include, as well as initial relative powerlessness of users of services, professional fears of loss of status and power, fear of change, lack of organisational support and lack of trust on the part of both users and professionals (Braye and Preston-Shoot, 1995). The existence of such a legacy means that changing practice will not be easy. However, the National Health Service and Community Care Act 1990 created the internal market for health care which created the scope for expression of individual choice, as well as the imperative of contracting for the health needs of the local population. Health service users have been given consumer status. The Government launched the 'Local Voices' initiative in 1992, urging health authorities to involve local people in their purchasing activities. The reforms of the National Health Service initially defined district health authorities as purchasers of health care; this responsibility now also falls on fund-holding general practitioners. While health authorities have overall responsibility for assessing the health care needs of the local population and for developing strategies to meet those needs, there is concern surrounding representation at this level. Health authorities are staffed by non-elected people. Since the implementation of the National Health Service and Community Care Act 1990 local council nominees, who previously represented the local communities, are no longer members of health authorities. These authorities consist of appointed members, and while there are non-executive directors, they are not required to represent all sectors the local community (Cooper *et al*, 1995; Smaje, 1995).

Unlike health authorities, community health councils do have some community representation. Half of their members are appointed by the local councils, one third by the voluntary sector and the rest by the health regions. They are entitled to be consulted on substantial developments or variations in service.The responsibilities of the community health councils have been expanded since 1991 and now include working closely with purchasers in identifying local needs, developing purchasing strategies and monitoring services. Community health councils, however, are poorly funded and have not been given additional resources to cope with their expanded responsibilities (Cooper *et al,* 1995). If health service users have been given consumer status, then they need to be involved in the planning of policies and services. Such activity is greater than being aware of the rights to health care which were explained in the Patients' Charter, which aimed to empower individual consumers of services. However, some individuals will be better able to articulate, claim and enforce their rights than others and it is important, within a caring context, to recognise this: a situation of relatively scarce health resources places responsibility on health professionals when it comes to providing an equitable service. This situation, of relations between people and the state being recognised in terms of transactions between individuals and the relevant state agency, leads Coote (1992) to question the scope for activities by groups of citizens whose interests may be better protected by working together rather than individually.

Abel-Smith *et al* (1995) describe how there are three principal means of involving the public in the development of health policies:

1. Through the representative democratic process

2. Through organised interest groups

3. Through direct involvement of individual citizens.

Barnes and Walker (1996) describe two models of user involvement.The consumerist model offers users a choice between products as service users 'shop around' individually seeking to satisfy their own needs without necessarily referring to others with similar needs. Alternatively, the empowerment model involves users in the development, management and operation of services as well as in the assessment of need. Barnes and Walker argue that this model allows users to identify collective interests and thus develop a collective position which enables fair treatment of all, not confined to current service users but also fair to citizens in general. Beresford and Croft (1993) describe the first steps to involvement as information gathering, often involving the use of surveys, and consultation, which implies a more interactive process. Secondly they identify the need to move towards people having a direct say in decision-making. However, Cooper *et al* (1995) state that in practice initiatives in response to 'Local Voices' are almost entirely at the level of consultation. Service user involvement does not necessarily lead to empowerment: there is a need to change the power balance in decision-making (Braye and Preston-Shoot, 1995).

Beresford and Croft (1993) describe involving people as a political activity comprising eight elements:

1. Resources are required as involving people needs time, space, skill and support, all of which will have financial implications.

2. Information is a prerequisite for people who make decisions about services.

3. Training is necessary both for providers and users of services as new skills and values prevail in a participative relationship.

4. Research and evaluation are essential to monitor the progress and effectiveness of participative programmes.

5. Equal access and opportunities are essential if people are to become equal partners in service provision.

6. Forums and structures need to be set up that foster involvement.

7. The language that is used needs to be one that empowers people rather than one that reflects or perpetuates inequalities.

8. Finally, Beresford and Croft conclude that advocacy is central to any discussion of involvement and empowerment, particularly self-advocacy where people articulate their own needs and rights either individually or collectively.

However, Barnes and Wistow (1992) warn against being dismissive of initiatives that seem modest in scope, as initiatives which appear to operate at the level of consultation may have a longer term effect of enhancing user empowerment as a result of involvement in unforeseen ways. For example, Beresford and Croft (1993) cite evidence of a disabled woman developing skills and confidence from getting involved in meetings and working with other people. Barnes and Walker (1996) have also identified that people can be empowered through their identification with others. People who are brought together as a consultation exercise can increase their confidence and ability to articulate their views as they work with others. This sort of participation may foster a synergistic effect.

The sum of a series of feasible incremental changes may be greater than a more radical initiative which fails through over-ambition

(Barnes and Wistow, 1992, p4).

Empowerment, thus, can be viewed as a process or as an outcome. The empowerment process enables people to make the connection between their private troubles and public policy by influencing and changing values and attitudes in policy and practice (Beresford and Croft, 1993). This process involves three elements, according to Beresford and Croft. Firstly people need to be able to talk about their experiences and recognise the possibility of articulating their concerns – 'developing their own accounts'. Secondly people need to 'form their own judgements' by deciding what changes are desirable and what is necessary to achieve them. These two stages can facilitate the move from feeling powerless to feeling more powerful. Thirdly, people need to 'negotiate with others' as it is not to be assumed that everyone in the same position will agree. In order to be effective, disparate community interests need to be coordinated to form a coherent position. Communities, which are only occasionally organised into interest groups, thus need to create organisational form, new concepts and language (Barker, 1996). A similar model is also proposed by Dalrymple and Burke (1995) in which the three stages are called biography, changed consciousness and political action. The outcome, then, of empowerment is positive self-esteem, the ability to set and reach goals, a sense of control over life and change processes and a sense of hope for the future (Rodwell, 1996).

In an attempt to address the methods used to involve people in planning and evaluating services, Barnes and Wistow (1992) conducted an evaluation of a Birmingham-based community care special action project. Three central questions were asked:

1. Which 'users' are involved?

2. How are people involved?

3. What is the outcome of involving users?

In terms of which users are involved, it is not always easy to attract participants who are representative of the community concerned. For example, when it was decided that it was no longer possible to offer a full range of state health care in Oregon, USA, a commission of professional and lay people was set up to prioritise conditions requiring health care. Various interest groups were consulted, telephone questionnaires were conducted and public meetings were held in order to involve the community in this decision making. However, Bowling (1992) reports that one problem with the meetings arranged to achieve community participation was that those who attended were not necessarily representative of the users of state health care, in that they were largely college educated, Caucasian, in high income groups, medical students and health professionals. Tomlin (1992) reports on an attempt by City and Hackney health authority to gain information from people in Hackney on what they saw as priorities for health care. While about fifty people were expected to attend a public meeting, only two people turned up, both middle-aged men – a mature student and a management consultant and thus not representative of the population of this area of east London. However, this must not be allowed to become an excuse for not involving people. When it comes to involving members of minority ethnic groups Beresford and Croft (1993) argue that it is essential to make specific provision to involve such people, as experience suggests that they do not become involved in general initiatives. Equal opportunities initiatives are needed that focus on ensuring that barriers to access services are removed; information provided for groups which are under represented needs to be in accessible formats (Braye and Preston-Shoot, 1995).

Many attempts are being made to involve users of services. Cooper *et al* (1995) describe research carried out by the Institute for Public Policy Research in 1994, which involved interviews with health authority officials and other relevant participants in decision making in England. It was found that information was sought from a variety of sources, for example, random representative samples, stratified samples, minority groups, voluntary organisations, special interest groups and users of specific services. Many different aspects of health care were addressed, including the location of a health centre, developing specific services, needs assessment and evaluating existing services.

In terms of how people are involved, the *Health for All* (WHO, 1992) strategy has emphasised the importance of communities promoting their own health and participating in decision making. Ong and Humphris (1994) argue that this philosophy has stimulated growth in community participation in projects in the health field. Ong and Humphris describe the 'rapid appraisal' method of needs assessment, which involves working in the field and learning directly from local inhabitants. Information collection is the result of an exchange between communities and professionals. 'Rapid appraisal' focuses on a community's own perspective of need, thus community involvement is central to this approach. Service providers need to gain access to communities and identify key informants who are knowledgeable about the community's problems, for example, community leaders. Qualitative interviews can then reveal rich data which will supplement epidemiological and demographic data. Once the information is obtained and analysed, areas of concern that have been identified can be referred to the community in order that they can determine priorities for action and assist in drawing up plans to address these concerns.

Further examples of how users can be involved can be found in outreach work, locating services closer to where people live and work. Another example of involving users of services can be found in the work of Hine *et al* (1995) which has already been referred to in this volume. This study aimed to find ways of promoting physical activity in south Asian women in the Bristol area. Partnership was ensured by a joint initiative involving the local Asian women's network, the health authority, sports development officers and the university.

What then is the outcome of involving users? Possible outcomes include a sense of ownership of initiatives to improve health, breaking down of barriers that may exist between providers and users of services, and the establishment of continuing dialogue and debate. Valuable networks can be established which may bring rewarding relationships for all parties involved. Arguably, most important is the sense of satisfaction that may be felt by both providers and users of services.

Empowerment of both communities and individuals should be an important part of policies that aim to tackle inequalities in health

(Benzeval, Judge and Whitehead, 1995, p110).

In attempting to raise awareness of issues of culture and discrimination this book aims to prepare health professionals for the reality of practice in a world where there is considerable geographical mobility, a reality to which they might aspire as professionals or as part of a family unit. While it is not possible to learn about all cultures, the preceding chapters should have provided a framework for learning about any group.

The text has taken an approach that focuses on similarities rather than emphasising differences. Although it is acknowledged that failure to have cultural needs met can be a problem for the individual and family, cultural diversity in itself is not a problem. The presence of a variety of ethnic groups and cultures in any society adds a richness and affords many benefits to that society. Art, literature, food, music and dance are just a small part. Learning and experiencing different values systems, social codes and religious and philosophical ideas challenges the *status quo* and offers alternative and refreshing ways of living our lives. Increasing interest and knowledge about the health care practices of other cultures is adding a holistic and generally safer dimension to western health care. The practices deemed backward by western medicine have the capacity not just to complement conventional health care but to replace many of the human qualities that have been lost.

References

Abel-Smith B, Figueras J, Holland W *et al* (1995) *Choices in Health Policy. An Agenda for the European Union.* Dartmouth, Aldershot

Barker C (1996) *The Health Care Policy Process.* Sage, London

Barnes M, Wistow G (eds.) (1992) *Researching User Involvement.* Nuffield Institute for Health Services Studies, Leeds

Barnes M, Walker A (1996) Consumerism versus empowerment: a principled approach to the involvement of older service users. *Policy and Politics.* 24(4)

Behrens R (1993) Managing diversity. *Viewpoint. The Magazine for Benefits Agency Managers.* **8:** 19

Behrens R, Auluck R (1993) *Action Planning for Diversity Management: a Comparative Perspective.* HMSO, London

Benzeval M, Judge K, Whitehead M (eds.) (1995) *Tackling Inequalities: An Agenda for Action.* King's Fund, London

Beresford P, Croft S (1993) *Citizen Involvement. A Practical Guide for Change.* Macmillan, London

Bowling A (1992) Setting priorities in health: the Oregon experiment. *Nursing Standard,* **6**(37): 29–32

Bray S, Preston-Shoot M (1995) *Empowering Practice in Social Care.* Open University Press, Buckingham

Cooper L, Coote A, Davies A, Jackson C (1995) *Voices Off. Tackling the Democratic Deficit in Health.* IPPR, London

Coote A (ed.) (1992) *The Welfare of citizens. Developing New Social Rights.* IPPR/Rivers Oram Press, London

Dalrymple J, Burke B (1995) *Anti-Oppressive Practice. Social Care and the Law.* Open University Press, Buckingham

Gibson CH (1991) A concept analysis of empowerment. *J Adv Nurs* **16:** 354–61

Hine C, Fenton S, Hughes AO, *et al* (1995) Coronary heart disease and physical activity in South Asian women: local context and challenges. *Health Education Journal.* **54:** 431–43

Kandola B (1993) Managing diversity. *Viewpoint. The Magazine for Benefits Agency Managers.* **8:** 18

Leathard A (ed.) (1994) *Going Inter-professional. Working Together for Health and Welfare.* Routledge, London

Mason D, Jewson N (1992) 'Race', equal opportunities policies and employment practices; reflections on the 1980s, prospects for the 1990s. *New Community.* **19**(1): 99–112

Ong BN, Humphris G (1994) Prioritizing needs with communities. Rapid appraisal methodologies in health. In: Popay J, Williams G eds. *Researching the People's Health.* Routledge, London

Pietroni P (1994) Inter-professional team-work: its history and development in hospitals, general practice and community care (UK). In: Leathard A ed. *Going Inter-professional. Working Together for Health and Welfare.* London: Routledge

Rodwell CM (1996) An analysis of the concept of Empowerment. *J Adv Nurs.* **23**: 305–13

Smaje C (1995) *Health, 'Race' and Ethnicity. Making sense of the Evidence.* King's Fund Institute, London

Tomlin Z (1992) Their treatment in your hands. Guardian. 29.4.92. p21

World Health Organisation (1992) *Targets for Health for All. The Health Policy for Europe. Summary of the Updated Edition September 1991.* WHO, Copenhagen

INDEX

A

abortion 131
acceptability of smoking 138
acceptance 199
access 55
access to health care 140
access to power x
accidents 7, 143
accommodation 132
acculturation enabler guide 181
active citizenship 24
active participation 147
activity at work and leisure 72
activity level 89
admissions 139
advocacy 64, 213, 217
affirm their identity 62
affirming belief 147
afro-caribbean 44
age x
ageism 52, 61
Ahmad 1, 3, 18
alcohol 72, 137
alcohol consumption 136
alcohol-related 138
Allen 4
Alleyne 4
altruism 21
ambivalent attitudes to
  emigration 136
ancillary workers 50
ante-natal care 143
Anthias 71
anti-discriminatory vii
anti-irish racism 136
anti-oppressive practice 62, 175

anti-racism 3, 212
anti-racist policies ix
anxiety 144
appropriate services 2
appropriateness 201
Arber and Ginn 45
arranged 129
Arthritis 133
asbestos 138
Asian 44
assessment skills 204
assimilation 45, 126
asthma 82
Asylum and Immigration Act
  (1996) 156
asylum-seekers ix,152
audit commission's 10
auxiliary nursing 50
availability of beds 144

B

back injury in nurses 133
Bahl 8
Balarajan and Bulusu 134
Bangladeshi 6
bankruptcy 99
Barbadian 47
Barton and Brown 177
Baxter 1
behaviour 136
Beishon 4
beliefs 53
belonging 44, 126
Berry 2
Beveridge Report 28

Beveridge Report on Social Insurance and Allied Services published in 1942 20
Bey 202
bill of rights 24
biological factors 1
biomedical 52
biomedical approaches 137
black african 6
black caribbean 6
Black Report 30
Blakemore 44
Blakemore and Boneham 47
blind backtranslation 167
blindness 53
blood cholesterol 80
Body Mass Index 76
born in Ireland 127
Bosnian refugees 158
Bosnians189
Bouri 108
British colonial system 47
Brown and Harris 103
Bruni 4
buffering 56

C

cancers 7, 138
Cardiff 48
caring. 177
case studies 6
cataract 54
catering 50
centrality of racism x
cervical smear 107
challenging prejudice 207
changing social values 145
Charter 88 24
chinese 6
chiropody 64
christianity 47
cirrhosis of the liver 139
citizen right 147
citizen rights 148
Citizen's Charter 7,25
citizenship xi, 18
citizenship and nationality 28
citizenship and social class 20
citizenship status 18
civic duties 21

class 46, 75
cleaning 50
client ix
client power 147
clinical skills 206
clothing industry 82
collaboration 8
collaborative partnerships 63
colonial ideologies of 'race' 49
commercial occupations 48
commision for racial equality x, 147
Commission on Social Justice 28
commissioning agencies 147
communication 9
community 8
community care 58
community development 168
community health councils ix, 215
community outreach 64
community participation ix, 219–20
concept analysis 176
concerned about being abandoned 60
condoms 114
confidante 58
congenital malformation 143
consangunity 143
Constantinides 71, 74
contraception 131
contribution 51
control over stressful aspects 138
Convention Relating to the Status of Refugees 1951 153
co-residence 57
coronary heart disease 7, 137
Cortese 12
Cortis 14
crisis intervention 62
Croats 188
cultural and religious traditions 130
cultural bereavement 135
cultural competence 62,177
cultural diversity vii
cultural health beliefs 194
cultural heterogeneity 44
cultural homogeneity xi

cultural knowledge 10
cultural meaning 53
cultural relativism 12
cultural sensitivity 64
cultural variations 2
culturalist approach 3
culturally competent skills xii
culturally sensitive 138
culturally sensitive care 14
culturally sensitive services 141
culture 2 ,52
culture shock 135
Cypriotness 103
Cyprus 73

D

Dalrymple and Burke 179
damage self identity xii
day service 59
Delphi Survey 9
demand 59
demographic data 69
denial 99
dental disorders 54
dependence 61
depression 82,143, 144
devaluation of old age 51
developmental screening 143
diabetes 53
diagnostic skills 204
diaspora 129
diet 85
diet and insulin 53
dietary habits 83
dignity 64
direct discrimination 209
disability 52– 53
disabled 8
disadvantage 44, 139
discrimination 2, 39, 44, 125, 142
discriminatory practices 1
disillusionment 47
diversity 46
division of land 128
divorce 127, 131, 133
domestic abuse 143
domestic disharmony 146
domestic service 130
dominant culture 177

double jeopardy 51
Dougherty 4
drug and alcohol abuse 145
drug use 141
drunkenness 139
dusty conditions 49

E

Ebrahim 52
economic and social
   marginalisation 142
economic deprivation 49
education 1
educational and occupational
   qualifications 135
efficiency 8
egalitarianism 26
elder abuse 60
elderly 8
Eleftheriadou 196
emigration 129
empathy 195
Empire Windrush 48
employment 75, 131
employment patterns 127
empowerment 178, 214
Enfield 70
Enfield and Haringey Health
   Authority 70
epidemiological 6
equal access 6
equal opportunities 39
equity 8,165
Eritrean 163
esponsiveness 8
ethical responsibility 14
ethnic conflict 188
ethnic group 6
ethnic identity 136
ethnic minority1
ethnicism 197
ethnicity 2,46,125
ethnocentric attitudes 140
ethnocentricity 2, 55
European Convention on Human
   Rights 153
European Union's Social
   Charter 23
eviction 143
evil eye 180

exceptional leave to remain 155
excluded xi
Exclusion xi
Expectations 140
Explanations for inequalities in
   health 31
exposure to cancer 138
expressing emotions 145
extended family 59
external control 136

F

family 57, 72
family at home 51, 129
family planning 143
Farooqi 196
Faulty equipment 132
fear of crime 57
feel inferior 144
femur fractures 54
Fernando 2
first generation 73
fitness status 77
focus groups 6
Folkman and Lazarus 100
follow-up appointment 140
food 72
Foolchand 13
foot 54
Francis *et al* 4
front-line 141

G

gender x, 52
gender and migration 129
genetic predisposition 144
George and Millerson 74
Gilbert 191
Ginn and Arber 26
good practice 63
GP consultations 104
Greek Cypriots xi
Greek Orthodox Church 74
Greek widows 187
Greekness 103
Greeks and Greek Cypriots 69
grief 128
guilt 140
Gujurat 47

H

halal f ood 53
Hanim 202
Haringey 70
heads of household 127
health 1,52
health behaviour xii
health belief model 33
health care 1
Health Education Authority 95
health of Irish 134
health patterns 134
health problems 112
health promotion 165
health screening 107
health status 143
health variations 69
health visitors 207
healthy behaviours 79
hearing impairment 54
heart disease 53, 80, 81
Heathrow Debate 9
Helman 102
heredity 134
heritage 62
heterogeneity 130
hierarchy of oppression 126
high-risk levels 139
Hinduism 47
Hindus 185
HIV/AIDS7 141
Hokanson Hawks 176
holocaust 190
home 46
home community 47
homeland 47
homeless x
homogeneity 46, 126
households 48
housing 31, 47
housing corporation x
housing status 133
housing status 132
human rights 188
hypertension 53, 80

I

identity 44, 57
illness 52
Immigration Act 50

immunisation 143
inappropriate diagnostic
   labelling 139
included xi
inclusion xi
income 51
Indian 6
indigenous 49
indigenous labour 49
indigenous population ix
indirect discrimination 209
individualised xi
individualised care 2
inequalities 52
inequalities in health xi, 30
infant mortality 143
informal care 59
informed choices 63
intellectualisation 99
intergenerational projects 61
interpersonal relationships 146
invisible Irish 126
Irish xi, 47, 125
Irish category in the census 147
Irish culture 140
Irish in Ireland 134
Irish professionals 137
Irish Republic 130
Irishness 140
Islam 47
isolation 134

J

Jamaican 47
Jamdagni 1
jews 48
job market 50
Johnson and Webb 175
justice 177

K

Kalisch 195
Karmi 5
Kavanagh and Kennedy 12
Kemp 177
key informants 166
King's Fund 10
kiria 203
kirios 203
kiritz and moos 103
kristallnacht 191

Kurdish refugees 162
Kushnick 5

L

labelling 176
labour market 47
language 6
language barriers 59
language differences 125
Leddy and Pepper 14
Leininger 3
leisure pursuits 61
life expectancy 51
life satisfaction 51
lifestyle 54, 69, 136, 140
linguistic 62
literacy 143
literature 1 28
Littlewood 100
liver damage 139
Liverpool 48
living alone 57
living arrangements 47
local authorities 8
Local Voices 215
locality 47
loneliness 134
loneliness and isolation 97
long term 53
longevity 45
long-term disability 132
long-term illness 81
loss of status 158
low birth weight 143
low class position 135
low income 136
low paid 132
low self-esteem 140
low worth xii
lower expectations 52

M

Maastricht Treaty 29
maintaining links 146
Maketon 11
mammogram 107
managing diversity 214
marginalisation ix
marital or filial relationship 60
marital status 127
marriages 129

Marshal 119
material deprivation 30
McMahon and Pearson 11
McNaught 108, 207
medical autonomy ix
mediterranean diet 85
mental illnes 7, 55,143
mental illness in Ireland 144
midwives 207
migrants ix
migration 44, 135
migration to America 128
minority ethnic groups 26
minority ethnic in-patient
    admissions 147
mobility 129
mode of transmission 141
model for transcultural care xii
Mohammed 7
monitoring 126
morbidity 53
mortality rates 52, 134
mother country 47
motivation 90
Multicultural 1
multiculturalism 212
multiculturalist ix
multiethnic 1
multiracial 1
Murphy and Macleod-Clark 10
muslims 185
myocardial infarction 80
myth of return 60

N
Nabarro 81
NAHA 5
National Health Service
    ix, 50, 131
National Health Service &
    Community Care Act 1990
    215
nationality 6
nazis 189
necrotic bone condition 133
needs assessment 6
negative stereotypes 146
neighbourhoods 47
New Commonwealth
    immigrants 100

new managerialism x
new pattern of emigration 131
NHS reforms x
Ni Bhrolochain 126
non-executive directo 147
Northern Ireland 130
nurse 130
nurses 131
nursing 9, 132
nursing models 11
nursing process 9
nursing students 50

O
Oakley 74
obligation 59
occupational groups 131
occupational injury 132
official sites 142
old age as a 'leveller 51
Oliver and Heater 21
oppression of a patriarchal
    society130
Oregon 219
orthodox jews 185
osteomalacia 54
other minorities 148
outreach 140
overweight 54

P
Pakistani 6
Parikiak 85
participating community xi
participation xi, 62
Paschalis 74
passive recipients 64
passivity 61
Patient's Charter 7, 25
patterns of migration 128
payment in kind 63
Pearson and Vaughan 11
Pederse 12
peer pressure 140
pensions 51
perceptions 53
persecution 48
persistence 137
personality disorders 144
persuasion 49
physical fitness 78

plans to return 61
Plant and Barry 18
pluralistic xi
political asylum
 questionnaire 154
political invisibility 126
poor housing 55, 136
poor nutrition 139
post war economy 48
poverty 4, 26, 55
power 176
prayer 145
prejudices 3
premature death 143
premature mortality 134
pre-retirement age/band 134
pressure to achieve 146
prevention of disease xi
primary care 106, 177
private medicine 105
private rented sectors 132
process of colonialism 144
professional and clinical
 freedom ix
professional education vii
professionals 39
professionals are socialise 146
promotion of health xi
Protocol relating to the status
 of Refugee 1967 155
public 132
public accountability ix
pull 49, 128
push 49

Q

qualitative studies 6
questionnaire 71

R

race 2
Race Relations Act 1976 208
racial discrimination 28
racial harassment 55,209
racism ix, 2 ,47, 52
Raleigh *et al* 53
Ramadan 53, 185
random sample 87
rapid appraisal 220
Rastafarians 185
rates of admission 144

RCN 11
recipe approach 186
recruiters 49
reduce harm 140
redundancy 99
Refugee 152
Refugee Arrivals Project 155
Refugee Council 162
Refugee Development
 Project 167
refugees ix, 177
relationship between suicide,
 socio-economic status and
 immigration 145
religion 6
religious 57
religious beliefs 56
religious groups 62
religious life 130
relocation 56
reminiscence activities 61
renal failure 53
repression 99
repressive religious attitudes 145
research 13, 52, 166
resources 63
respiratory 137
responsibility for caring 60
retired 131
rheumatism 133
rights 63
rish economy 128
risk factors 81
Roman Catholic 189
Roper9
Rosenbaum 182
Rosenhan 176
Royal College of Physicians 92
rural communities 131

S

safe sex 141
safety provision 132
salt 54
Sands and Hale 4
sanitation 143
schizophrenia 144
screening 106
second generation 73, 137
second class citizens 26

selective provision 22
self esteem 51
self reports 52
semi-skilled48
semi-structured interviews 87
sense of worthlessness 145
Serbs 188
servant 48
service contracts 213
sexual health 7, 113
sexual identity 141, 146
shared meanings 52
sheltered housing 59
sickle cell disorde 34
sickness benefit 133
Sikh women 58
Sikhism 47
similarities and variations 193
skilled professional 48
skin cancer 138
skin colour 49, 125
Slaves 48
Slovens 188
Smaje 3, 197
smoking 72, 136
snowball sample 87
social activities 101
social and cultural determinants1
social class x, 51
social cohesion 30
social justice 37
social life 72
social mobility 135
social networks 133
social roles 57
social selection 134
social stigma of remaining
    single 130
social support 51, 146
social support networks 57
socially isolated 133
socio-economic factors 137
sociology of ageing 45
Somali 163
spiritual resources57
sporadic employment 132, 136
staff 64
standard acknowledgment
    letter 154
Star of David 191

State Enrolled Nurse 50
State Registered Nurse 50
statistical data 147
statistical invisibility 126
Steenbergen21
Steinberg and Sykes 93
stereotype 125
stereotypes 5
stigma 55, 141
stigmatisation xii
stillbirth 143
Stockwell 175
stomach ulcers 139
strategic planning 63
stress 54, 72, 96, 135
stress reducers 97
stroke7, 54
structural factors 136
Stubbs 5
stupid stereotype 131
subjective experience 52
suicide 145
Sumner 2
support for travellers142
surveys 6
sweat shops 82

T

targets for health for all 165
teacher 130
textile industry 49
thalassaemia 34, 69
the past 128
Theodorou 87
theories of health 134
theory of human capital 33
third generation & other 73
Thomas 10
three generation households 57
tied accommodation 132
tobacco 136
tolerated 142
Torkington 1 ,4
total abstainers 139
trade unions 138
traditions 44
transcultural education 5
transcultural model 62
transcultural nursing 2
transient 139

transport 55
travellers 142
triple jeopardy 51
Tripp-Reimer 4
Tschudin 195
Tuberculosis 31, 55, 137, 164
Turkish culture 184

U

UKCC 13
UN High Commission for
   Refugees 153
understand i, 53
unemployed x, 132
unemployment 26, 145
unhealthy behaviours 80
uniformity 126
United Nations 153
Universal Declaration of Human
   Rights 153
universal provision 22
unpopular patients 175
unskilled 48
unskilled workers 131
upkeep of the family 129
use of accident and
   emergency 104
user 39
user involvement 216
users 7

V

van Dijk 197
vegans 185
victim-blaming 10, 32
victimisation 209
visited at home 140
visual impairment 54
voluntary sector 63
volunteering 103
vulnerable people 8

W

walking problems 54
ways of coping 52
Weinman 103
welfare rights 59
well-being 51
white 6
white-collar jobs 131
widowed 127

widowhood 133
widows 58
Wilding 176
women 51, 132
work profile 98
working collaboratively with
   professionals 147
World Health Organisation 180

Y

Yugoslavia 188